DATE			

From Here to Maternity

From Here to Maternity

Confessions of a
First-Time Mother

Carol Weston

Little, Brown and Company
Boston   Toronto   London

First Edition

Excerpt from "The Long Boat" by Stanley Kunitz from *Next-to-Last
Things*. Copyright © 1985 by Stanley Kunitz. Used by permission of
Atlantic Monthly Press.

Excerpt from "All I Really Need" by Raffi, D. Pike, B. & B. Simpson.
Composer: Raffi. Copyright © 1980 by Homeland Publishing, a divi-
sion of Troubadour Records Ltd. Used by permission of Troubadour
Records Ltd.

Library of Congress Cataloging-in-Publication Data

Weston, Carol.
    From here to maternity : confessions of a first-time mother /
Carol Weston. — 1st ed.
        p.   cm.
    ISBN 0-316-93163-2
    1. Pregnancy. 2. Childbirth. 3. Weston, Carol. 4. Mothers—
United States — Biography.   I. Title.
RG525.W57   1991   90-19853
618.2'4 — dc20

                    10   9   8   7   6   5   4   3   2   1
                                    FG

Published simultaneously in Canada by Little, Brown & Company
(Canada) Limited

Printed in the United States of America

Dedicated to
my daughter Elizabeth
and
my mother, Mary Elizabeth

Contents

Acknowledgments

With heartfelt thanks to all the family and friends who encouraged me along the way, and to those who read and critiqued early drafts of this book: Dr. Stephanie Bird, Hannah Duncan, Janet Goldstein, Cathy Roos, Bernadette Anthony, Michelle Ganon, Carol Morton, Heidi Greene, and Cynthia Weston. With still more thanks to my mother and mother-in-law and all the others who went above and beyond the call of duty by not only critiquing the book but by letting themselves be characters in it: Patty, Susan, Ed, Beth, Seth, Lucie, and Leslie. (I won't blow their covers now.) With even more thanks to my husband, whose cover was blown long ago and who was nonetheless willing to read and reread. I am also grateful to my indefatigable agent, Connie Clausen, my wonderful and incredibly thorough editor, Fredrica Friedman, her terrific assistant, Becky MacDougall, and painstaking project copy editor David Coen. And to Amy, who helped me start, and Emme, who let me finish. And finally to Ursula K. Le Guin, whom I don't know, for having written in a *New York Times Book Review* article entitled "The Hand That Rocks the Cradle Writes the Book":

> The difficulty of trying to be responsible, hour after hour, day after day, for maybe twenty *years*, for the well-being of children and the excellence of books, is immense. . . . And we don't know much about the process, because writers who are mothers haven't talked much about their motherhood — for fear of boasting? for fear of being

trapped in the Mom trap, discounted? . . . It seems to me a pity that so many women, including myself, have accepted this denial of their own experience . . . writing as if their sexuality were limited to copulation, as if they knew nothing about pregnancy, birth, nursing, mothering. . . . To have and bring up kids is about as immersed in life as one can be, but it does not always follow that one drowns. A lot of us can swim.

Introduction

I was great with child. Strangers on the street congratulated me, wished me good luck, asked me when I was due. "Two weeks!" I'd answer with a pride and contentment that surprised even me.

I passed women carrying briefcases. I passed women carrying babies. And I realized at last how much I was looking forward to putting down my pencils and picking up my newborn. I still had projects to finish, yet at times I could hardly wait for the birth day.

When I massaged my belly, I was already cradling my baby. When the baby shifted, I tried to press my hands against his or hers. Each kick was a hello from the future. Sometimes I talked or sang to my child-to-be. Sometimes I just tried to picture the little being that was about to turn my life upside down.

Was it a boy or a girl? Would he or she arrive easily? Would I know how to comfort, to nurse, to mother? How would my marriage and friendships change?

I knew that many babies were colicky, that not all were born normal. I knew motherhood was not a Mary Cassatt painting. Yet sometimes I put my arms around my enormous belly and felt as serene as a smiling Buddha. I had to believe that inside me a beautiful child was blossoming.

Two weeks. My husband now jumped when I phoned him at work. Our mothers both considered themselves on call. And friends were checking in more than ever. We were all waiting for the baby — to have and to hold and to love.

Part One

Womb Service

Rob talked me into it.

"I don't get it," he said as we shared an ice-cream cone on West End Avenue. "What are we waiting for?"

"I'm just not ready."

"When will you be ready?"

"I don't know."

We were in the middle of a baby boomlet, and many of my friends — married and unmarried — were obsessed by babies. They'd stop at every stroller, coo at every Snugli.

Not me. As a teen, I baby-sat until I had baby-sitter burnout. I knew kids were work. I also knew that once you had children — and no longer had time — your life lurched into fast forward.

Trouble was, I liked my life. My husband, my home, my friends, my work. As a writer, I worked odd hours, all hours. I had lunches with editors. I went on book tours. Things were where I wanted them to be: I was a Dear Abby for teens and had a third book on the way. Teens, I felt, were interesting. Babies, I feared, were a bore.

"We don't even know if you're fertile," Rob said.

No, we didn't. But it killed me that my having been responsible, and never having gotten pregnant, could now be used against me. I hated being reminded that my thirty-year-old ovaries were not getting any younger.

"What if we have a problem?" he persisted.

"What if we have a baby?"

"It'll be great. We'll love it."

"The whole thing just scares me. It's going to change my life more than yours."

"You know I'll be a good father."

"I know you work long hours."

The nineties dad: sensitive, helpful, nurturing, never home.

He sighed. "You promised, remember?"

What I promised was that on New Year's Day the diaphragm would go out the window.

What happened was that on New Year's Day I panicked and begged for time.

"Just six more weeks," I pleaded. "We'll go wild on Valentine's Day. It'll be perfect! It'll be romantic!"

Yet on February 14, I clutched again. I'd never in my life made love without birth control. I felt pressured, confused, guilty. "I'm sorry. Next month, I swear. Ready or not. We'll do it in March."

I meant it, too. I was beginning to realize that I might never be ready. That there was no perfect time. That if I waited to catch the baby bug, I might wait forever. Part of me was even glad Rob was being insistent about this. Because I did want children. Had he been dead set against fatherhood, *I* might have been the one pushing babies. Maybe every couple needs one person to be adamant about the big issues.

But come March, I was still petrified — though also annoyed at myself for dragging my heels.

I guessed at my most fertile days and prayed Rob would have out-of-town business. He didn't. I feigned headaches and sleepiness and came up with creative ways of keeping him happy and me safe. I thought I was home free for another month.

No such luck. When we came home from dinner out and a movie starring Mel Gibson (my personal heartthrob), I reached into the medicine cabinet. "Don't bother," Rob said. "I don't even want to if we're not trying to make a baby. Really. What's the point?"

Withholding sex: the Lysistrata technique.

"Oh, c'mon," I said. We'd been married six years. Were we really going to have to argue recreation versus procreation?

"Listen, I mean it."

I protested.

I called him a bully.

I climbed into bed.

Rob folded me into his arms and kissed me. And there, beneath our blue-and-white quilt, with our cat purring at our feet, we did it. Tentatively, tenderly. For God and for country. And for us.

It still seems . . . inconceivable.

While Rob and I basked in lazy afterglow, those long-dormant pipes of mine chugged into action. My body not only knew sperm when it saw them, but went out of its way to make the little swimmers feel right at home.

"Gentlemen callers!" my eggs must have cried. "Catch them!"

In retrospect, I suppose I could say that our lovemaking that night felt extra special. That Rob's joyful contribution made me think somehow of shooting stars. That in some profound and, indeed, rather flaky way, I could almost trace the distance that one particular star was traveling, its long night's journey into day.

I could even confess that my husband often lights candles before we make love — candles I usually blow out afterward while Rob is asleep. This time, he lit the candles but we *both* fell asleep. I awoke with a start an hour later to find wax all over the table but, fortunately, no flames leaping about our bedroom.

Hindsight may be a fine detective, but back then I was clueless. I chalked up the stars and candle wax to steamy sex.

Naive, I know, but it just didn't occur to me that I might become pregnant that first night. I didn't think it would be so easy. We have friends who have been trying for years. And since I'd delayed childbirth in favor of my career — a large part of which has been spent telling teens *not* to get pregnant — I half expected some divine justice would make it hard for me to conceive.

Besides, my period (or lack thereof) was still many days away. And I felt no more tired than your average overworked, overwhelmed New Yorker. The notion that I was pregnant was so far from my mind that I didn't even think about renouncing coffee and alcohol — let alone postponing our annual spring ski trip.

Rob and I had planned a ski vacation in Utah with his parents and our friend Seth, whom I'd known since we were kids.

Actually, Seth had planned it. He knew he had a standing invitation to join us anytime, and as a med student, time was something he had little of. We'd talked about April in Park City, but Seth made it happen.

"I reserved three seats to Salt Lake City on April ninth," he told our answering machine. "TWA Flight 743. Are you game?"

Why not? We called Seth. We called TWA. We were off.

On the way to the airport, my husband, a.k.a. Mr. Discretion, announced that I was "knocked up."

"Seth, don't listen to him," I said. "I'm not even late yet."

"Knocked up," Rob repeated. "Mark my words."

We met my in-laws and skied all over Park City, Alta, Deer Valley, and Snowbird. We braved expert runs, sped over moguls, glided through bowls. I didn't fall any more than usual, but I did make a lot more pit stops.

This is how it worked. We'd hop off the gondola and I'd ask everyone to wait a minute. Then I'd take off my gloves, put down my poles, snap out of my skis, tromp off to the ladies' room, remove my parka, unzip my ski outfit, pull down my pants, sit down, stand up, pull up my pants, zip up my ski outfit, slip into my parka, tromp back to the slope, snap into my skis, put my gloves back on, and pick up my poles. And I'd be all set for, oh, thirty minutes or one run, whichever came first.

Too much hot chocolate at breakfast?

I didn't begin to catch on until the end of the third day. By then the hot tub outside was finally working, so we had all poured some wine, got into our bathing suits, made a run for it, and eased in. Ahhhh. Nothing like a hot tub on a cold day.

We sipped and we simmered; we simmered and we sipped. After about ten minutes, I started feeling overheated, so I hopped out to take a shower.

Next thing I knew, I was sitting naked on the floor of the shower stall. My head was propped against the wall and water was streaming down my face. I felt faint and queasy and it was all I could do to rinse off and get out of there.

Too much hot after too much cold?

Seth was reading in the kitchen.

"I feel really lightheaded," I said. "Do you think I could be pregnant?"

"I think you should sit down," said the doctor-to-be, and he brought me a tall glass of water.

Pregnant, I thought. And here I've been skiing and drinking and hot-tubbing — squashing and pickling and poaching my baby.

Pregnant? I wondered. And I resolved not to bomb down any more hard runs and not to sip or simmer for the rest of the trip.

Pregnant! I drank the cold water.

Stop here," Rob said to the taxi driver who had picked us up at Kennedy.

"Why?" I asked. We were still several blocks from home.

"I'm going to run in and get a pregnancy test."

"Honey, that can wait. Let's go home and check on the cat and open our mail and everything."

"I'll be back in two seconds," Rob said and ran into the pharmacy.

I smiled sheepishly at the driver, then slid back into the seat and looked out the window. A pregnant woman walked by holding hands with a tired toddler. A woman with a waist walked by holding hands with a good-looking man. I glanced at the driver for sympathy but noticed a snapshot of his little ones taped to the dashboard. What was I getting myself into?

Rob must not have bought the easiest kind of pregnancy test. The droppers and test tubes reminded me of high-school chemistry, and we both had to read the directions several times that night to figure out what we'd have to do the next morning.

My job, essentially, would be to donate some urine to the cause. Rob's would be to oversee the science lab, mixing and shaking and waiting the required thirty minutes for the results — a circle if I was pregnant, no change if I wasn't.

At 7:00 A.M. Rob nudged me. "Go for it," he said.

I groaned.

"If we don't do it first thing, we'll have to wait a whole 'nother day."

God forbid, I thought, and stumbled toward the bathroom.

For Rob, the wait proved interminable. He paced back and forth waiting for a circle to appear. I know fathers pace in maternity wards, but this was being overzealous, no? I pulled the covers over my head and tried to doze, sleep, buy time.

It was impossible. He hovered over the test like a kid waiting for a plant to grow. And he kept making announcements: "Nothing yet." "Still nothing." "No change." "Still nothing." And then, "Oh my God! Carol, a circle! A circle is forming! Buddy, you're pregnant!"

He pulled me out of bed, gave me a big hug, and started jumping all around. Sure enough, there by my soap and tooth-paste was a vial with a tiny telltale circle letting me know that my life was about to be rerouted and that I had better start drinking lots of milk.

I wished I could have felt as immediately ecstatic as Rob, but I don't live life at the intensity that he does. On a scale of one to ten, Rob often rates an eleven on enthusiasm. He's impulsive; I'm cautious. He leaps; I take baby steps. Pregnant? I was still coming to terms with trying to conceive. I'd need nine months to get used to the idea. And while I knew I was lucky it had happened so easily, I was also dazed.

We debated whether to take a photo of the circle and ulti-mately decided not to. "But get it all down in your journal," Rob said. Then he asked me what sign the baby would be.

Sign? As in zodiac?

I married this man of my own free will, I thought to myself.

"Sagittarius, just like you," I said aloud.

Rob was doubly pleased. He hummed a lot that day.

And he called to make a reservation at a nearby French restaurant.

Me? I called to make an appointment with my gynecol-ogist — whom I had just promoted to ob/gyn.

Over the next few days, the news, though still unofficial, began to sink in. It felt weird, but okay. I wondered if I might even be disappointed if the doctors didn't confirm our findings.

Drs. Yale and Romoff's waiting room was filled with big women and little kids. I gave one woman a knowing nod, but she looked at me puzzled, like: "What are you smiling at, skinny?" So I turned my attention to the rug rats: a girl with a hair bow, a boy with a missing tooth.

To my astonishment, I found myself getting choked up.

A child, I was going to have a child.

The receptionist called my name, requested a urine specimen, and pointed to the ladies' room. I went in, still stunned by the idea of really becoming a mom. Then I emerged. Empty-handed.

"Your specimen?" she asked. Specimen? I'd been too lost in thought to fool with paper cups. Boy, did I feel stupid.

"Don't worry," I said. "In about two minutes, I'll be able to try again."

Indeed, moments later I produced what they needed. The technician whisked it away, added some chemicals, and waited to see if a dot would appear. One did.

"Nice dot!" she exclaimed. "Great shade of blue."

"Can I see?" I asked.

They showed me my dot. I can't tell you how proud I felt of my dot. It was scary how proud I felt of my dot. I felt like crowing, "That's my dot!" I was ready to hand out cigars to the large ladies in the waiting room.

"You're pregnant all right," the technician assured me. "Is that good news?"

"Yes," I said, without a moment's hesitation.

Then, since we were just a few blocks from the Metropolitan Museum of Art, I said to my belly, "C'mon, kid, let's go get some culture." We headed to the Van Gogh exhibit. On the way, I smiled at every child and noticed buds opening on all the trees.

The surprise, I realized, was not that I was pregnant. The surprise was that it was indeed such good news.

You're supposed to wait at least ten weeks before spreading the word. We waited about ten minutes.

We started with parents. We figured parents would be easy. Parents would be happy.

Rob went to the kitchen and dialed Ohio. I found the cordless phone and was poised to pick up when his parents did.

"Mom, get Dad on the phone," Rob began. "We have very big news."

I waited until Rob's father said hello. "Remember how I almost fainted during our ski trip?" I asked.

"You're pregnant!" my mother-in-law screamed. "Congratulations! Oh, that's just great!" She had been wanting grandkids for years — particularly since her twin had pulled ahead three to nothing in the grandchild department. Gene has dedicated her life to teaching preschool. She adores kids, anybody's kids. And we weren't just anybody.

She immediately wanted to know how many months pregnant I was (one), how I was feeling (fine), and when was the due date (December 17). Rob's sister was about to have a baby in Boston, and two grandchildren on the way was almost more than Gene could handle. Her cup was overflowing. My guess is that she reached for her knitting needles as soon as we hung up.

Ken, my father-in-law, is not so effusive. A successful businessman, he's not the demonstrative type. Of course he was pleased that his only son was going to be a father. But what he said was: "Does this mean I'll have to sleep with a grandmother?" and "If it's born before New Year's, you'll get a tax deduction" and "Don't forget that we need a boy to carry on the family name."

After we signed off, I was half inclined to take a breather before making any more calls. After all, *I* was still getting used to

12

our news. But once you get the ball rolling, it's hard to slow it down.

We called my mother and invited her to dinner that night.

And my father? According to legend, one reason my mother married him was that when they were dating, she was charmed by how good he was with children. He *was* good. When we were younger, he played Crazy Eights and Scrabble with us, took us shopping for groceries and shoes, cooked our favorite foods: pork chops, turkey pot pie, and hamburgers ("But Daaad, no onions or fancy sauces, okay?").

He was proud of us, too. His eyes filled with tears when I published my first article in *Seventeen*, when I was graduated from college, and when we walked down the aisle together on my wedding day.

Dad was Santa Claus.

But Dad was dead.

Born in Russia in 1913, he died in Texas of a sudden heart attack in 1982. His death left a big hole in my life, and it took me a long time to learn to step around that hole without falling in. A long time before I could remember his laughter without feeling sad. Before I could enjoy his favorite things — Mozart, Shakespeare, Bing cherries, summer breezes — without missing him terribly.

I'd been the apple of his eye. Without Dad, it was hard for this daddy's girl to feel like much of an apple.

And it was hard to tell my father-in-law about my pregnancy when I wanted to tell my father.

I knew I was in for a new wave of missing him. Dad would have loved to have seen me pregnant, to have served me heaping platefuls of food and, down the road, to have tickled and teased a grandson or granddaughter. He might not have signed up for diaper-changing or round-the-clock baby-sitting, but he would have bounced his grandchildren on his knee as he had bounced me. He'd have shown off the baby photos. When they were old enough, he'd have even played monster with them. Because of a boyhood baseball accident, Dad's top front teeth were on a bridge, and when he felt mischievous, he could press the bridge a half inch forward and send us kids laughing and screaming in all directions.

A baby? Grandkids? Dad would have eaten them up.

He most certainly would have wanted to know. So I decided to tell him. Rob was making dinner, and I went into our room and sat up in bed.

"Dad?" I said. Was it softly or silently? "Dad? I'm pregnant." I looked at his photo on my night table. "I'm pregnant and you're going to live on in my child. I'm going to tell my baby about you and I'm going to show him pictures and you're going to be part of his life. He's going to know what he's missing, but also what he has of you."

I remembered saying good-bye to my father five years earlier, crying over his coffin in the funeral home about how much I'd miss him and how I appreciated everything he'd ever done for me and how I was so glad that I knew that he knew that I loved him and that nothing was left unsaid between us. I hadn't lifted the coffin lid because I hadn't wanted to see him with his eyes forever closed, and his mouth, according to my mother, set in a tight smile that wasn't his.

Even then I'd felt a little self-conscious.

Still, it had felt right to say good-bye.

Could I now say hello? I didn't know.

I wished I could believe that Dad could look out from the framed photos I have of him and see, not just that life goes on, but that *his* life would go on. That I was going to have a baby, a baby who would inherit his Russian blood and also, I hoped, his quick wit, gift for language, head for numbers, taste for wine, and love of *le mot juste*. If only Dad could be there for the first smile, first word, first step — I wanted him to know how welcome he'd be.

I touched his photo and said, "Look down on us if you can." Should I have said, "Look up"? Maybe. Dad had once joked that all the fun people would be in hell.

Telling my mother was delicate. My mother married a widower three years after my father's death, and the two of them were like newlyweds. They went to plays, movies, restaurants, parties, bed. They were passionate about each other — I was careful not to phone before nine *or* after nine. Sure, Mom would be delighted to have a grandchild, but I didn't know how she'd feel about being a grandmother.

My mother and Lewis were due any minute for dinner. It was a scene I'd rehearsed years ago. I'd lean forward, clasp my mother's hand, and whisper, "Robert and I are going to have a baby," at which point her eyes would mist and Rob would break out chilled champagne — which I wouldn't drink.

In reality, Mom and Lewis had scarcely walked in and lifted their martinis when Rob, irrepressible, said, "Guess who's got a bun in the oven?"

Mom clapped and Lewis toasted. But then for some reason, I got embarrassed and started backtracking and saying how it was awfully early to celebrate. Mom followed my retreat and agreed that we shouldn't count on things just yet. And next thing we knew, we were all thinking about miscarriages.

Instead of baby carriages.

My fault. I'd done the rain dance at this parade.

Yet while it worried me for our news to be greeted with unbridled celebration, it frustrated me for it to be greeted with sensible caution.

Apparently, saying you're pregnant is not like announcing a birth. It's happy news contingent on delivery of the goods nine months later.

The prudent thing to do would have been for Rob and me to keep quiet for another couple of months. The first is the riskiest trimester, and there was no need to hang up all the streamers and release all the balloons.

But we couldn't keep the excitement to ourselves.

That ball we'd gotten rolling? It was picking up speed.

Who else would we tell?

Grandparents. My granddad was ninety; Rob's was eighty. Our stepgrandmothers were right up there, too. Why save until tomorrow something they could enjoy today? We got Texas and Florida on the line.

Siblings next: his sisters, my brothers. Recently, whenever we'd left a message on their answering machines saying we had news, they'd call us back, all excited, and exclaim, "You're pregnant?" "No," we'd correct, feeling vaguely apologetic. Then we'd mumble something about a job or book contract or travel plan. This time we wouldn't let them down.

Finally, there were friends to consider, especially close friends, close by and close in age. Most had already been back and forth with me on the motherhood decision and would undoubtedly notice if I started ordering seltzer or milk, or if I started losing my waist and gaining a bust.

Still, did we really need to race through our Rolodex? What was the rush? And what if the fetus didn't "stick"?

"If something happened," Rob pointed out, "The first thing you'd do is get on the phone."

He was right. He would, too. We wouldn't want to go through the disappointment alone.

Ever since I was in junior high, my friends and I had discussed every setback — every broken nail, broken promise, broken heart. I still wasn't good at absorbing bad news on my own. The more I shared it, the more I accepted it.

I guess it was the same with happy news: the more Rob and I told people we were pregnant, the more we believed it.

Maybe we'd be telling them only to untell them, but what were friends for? The problem? If we told one friend, we'd have to tell them all. Our pregnancy was not something we wanted anyone close to learn secondhand.

17

We decided to exercise extreme willpower and managed to wait two more days before getting out the megaphone. Our poor confidants! In on this from week three. Mine was going to seem like the gestation period of an elephant.

None of our city friends were pregnant or had kids — which is one reason I hadn't felt I was being sluggish about birthin' babies. In New York, if you're thirty and childless, you fit right in. Here, millions of things scream for your attention; it's easy not to think about your biological clock.

Unless, of course, someone near and dear to you is thinking about hers. It's one thing to tell much younger couples or much older couples about being pregnant, but peers without kids have a stake in all this. We were about to make friends focus on something they might not want to focus on, and I had mixed feelings about stirring up mixed feelings. I don't know if I was being compassionate and sensitive or egocentric and neurotic, but I felt funny, for instance, about telling Beth and Ed.

We love Beth and Ed. They met in college in Wisconsin and went out for seven happy years. One day, while Ed was still waffling before the specter of commitment, Beth said, "Ed, I'm getting married this year. Are *you*?" He was. They married, moved to New York, got involved with nonprofit do-good careers, and started trying to have a family. They spoke to us glowingly about sex without birth control. They spoke to us lovingly about their nephews and nieces. And for two weeks each month, Beth abstained from drinking, in case she conceived. But months, then years, slipped by without event.

Along came Rob and his ambivalent wife. They give it one shot and bingo: Insta-baby. Of course I felt funny.

The four of us met for dinner at a Caribbean restaurant. Ed and Rob ordered beer. Beth and I ordered juice. We smiled at each other.

"I think I'm pregnant," I confessed.

"You think you're pregnant, or you *are* pregnant?" Beth asked.

"I am pregnant. We took the test."

"And it came out positive?"

"It came out positive."

They threw their arms in the air and whooped and hollered and said, "Congratulations!"

They didn't seem to be thinking, "She's pregnant; why aren't we?" They seemed delighted. But I still felt sheepish and hoped they'd have news of their own before I started knocking into things stomach-first.

Telling Susan and Miguel was awkward for a different reason. We'd had endless talks with them recently about parenthood, responsibility, insurance. About feeling older, feeling apprehensive, feeling ready. Then Susan got pregnant. Then Susan had a miscarriage. Now they were trying again, and though I knew it wasn't a race, I felt guilty beating them to the punch.

When we told them, they fussed and carried on, too. I said, "Hey, you'll make out like bandits because now *we'll* be lending *you* maternity clothes and baby outfits." An arrogant quip, I realized later. Who was to say my fetus wouldn't self-destruct?

The next day, Susan called to ask how I was feeling and said, "You know, I would have been five months along by now." I knew. And I was glad we could talk about it. It would have been worse to have become too careful of her feelings and to lose, in the name of courtesy, all sincerity and spontaneity.

That evening I called everyone else. I slipped into bed in my nightgown and knee socks with my cat, telephone, address book, and a tall glass of milk. Seth was jubilant (and hardly surprised). Valerie wasn't home. And when I reached my other female friends, they shrieked and cheered and made all the appropriate noises. But again — I'm crazy, I know — I worried about stepping on toes. Jen, my friend from sixth grade, and Meredith, my funny lawyer friend, and Patty, my novelist friend, wouldn't mind being married and pregnant themselves.

Did my news make them wistful? Was I somehow betraying them by taking this step forward and away?

Women's magazines warn that friendships can shift when a couple becomes a family. But I had to believe that my friendships were built on bedrock. That despite the underside of human nature, my friends wouldn't hold my pregnancy against me — or against themselves. If Patty got a Pulitzer Prize, I'd be thrilled, not jealous — wouldn't I?

Wouldn't I?

Maybe I'd be both. Maybe that's okay.

Valerie and I met for lunch at a Japanese restaurant. We'd known each other for over twenty years. In grade school, we slept at each other's houses; in college, we visited each other's dorms. Now we were both writers living in New York. But we were worlds apart. While I wrote for mainstream magazines like *Redbook* and *Ladies' Home Journal,* she wrote for hip publications like *Spy* and *Spin.* After all these years, I still dressed carefully when I went out with Val; I stayed on guard not to look like a fashion victim, a *Glamour* magazine "Don't."

I walked in and saw her at a corner table. Her curly blond hair set off dangling earrings. The dress code for diehard New Yorkers is to always look like you're on your way to a funeral, and Valerie was wearing black from head to toe.

"How are you?" she said, and put down her cigarette to give me a hug. "It's been a long time."

The waitress brought her a bottle of Kirin and asked if I'd like a drink. "Just cranberry juice." We looked over the menus and Val ordered sushi — which I love but which my pregnancy books said was off-limits. I ordered tempura.

"So what's new?" Val asked.

"I'm one-month pregnant," I said, deadpan.

Maybe Val misinterpreted my delivery, because her response seemed out of line.

She drew on her cigarette. "You can still do something about it."

I stared at her incredulous. "I wasn't totally ready beforehand, and I admit I wouldn't have minded waiting a few more months. But now that I'm pregnant, I'm psyched. My maternal instinct has kicked in."

"Oh. I'm sorry, I didn't mean — Listen, that's great. I think I'm just in shock."

It'd be a lie to say we ate in awkward silence. We didn't. We recovered quickly and gossiped away the lunch hour. But I wondered if the women's magazines were right. I wondered if the paths Val and I were choosing were beginning to drift further apart than our hands and hearts could stretch.

Abortion? I'd never considered abortion.

I wanted this baby. I was just finding out how much.

The next week I collected the teen mail from my post office box and settled down to answer it.

A twelve-year-old wrote,

My mom remarried three years ago. My stepdad's brother has a son, so he is my stepcousin. If we get married, will our kids turn out retarded?

No, but take things slowly, was my sage response. Frightening how early we women start worrying about the next generation!

A thirteen-year-old asked,

How do you French-kiss? My boyfriend and I have kissed but we haven't Frenched yet. I have the feeling he knows how, but I don't. So if you would write down the details of how French-kissing starts and ends and how to hold him during the process, it would be helpful. But I need the information very soon so please HURRY!!!

French-kissing: where it all begins. I sent her some pointers and assured her that inexperience is okay and that there was no need for it to appear that she'd perfected her technique on the whole soccer team.

A sixteen-year-old wrote,

I think I am pregnant and I am scared. My boyfriend lives 130 miles away. He said he would stand by me no matter what. But tonight he called and said he's starting to see other people. He doesn't have any right to leave me, does he? I don't believe in abortion and I am afraid to give up my baby. But I keep thinking I have the rest of my life ahead of me and I am afraid it is ruined. Please write me. I can't tell my parents — they'd kill me.

I get letters like this often, but that morning it struck me more clearly than ever how awful it would be to be pregnant

and alone, pregnant without fanfare, pregnant without someone who loved you and who wanted your baby as much as you
did. I wrote her a two-page reply filled with information and
advice. And I felt deeply thankful that, despite my initial ambivalence, my pregnancy was a reason to rejoice. My baby was
a wanted baby.

Then the ob/gyn's office called. "Have you heard the result of
your blood test?" asked Liz, a nurse I liked.

I went cold. "No, why?"

"Your progesterone level is low, so we'd like you to come in
for another test. It could be nothing."

"If it's *not* nothing, what could it be?"

"An ectopic pregnancy or a blighted ovum."

I had to ask.

Liz continued. "If it were an ectopic pregnancy, you'd probably have felt some pain."

"And if it's a blighted ovum?" I said in a half whisper.

"Just come in."

I knew an ectopic pregnancy meant a tubal pregnancy. But
what was a blighted ovum? I shoved the mail aside and got out
my dictionary. It defined blight as a plant disease. I checked the
indexes of my pregnancy books and found only bladder, bleed-
ing, blood, and the blues.

I got on the crosstown bus and considered the worst. I'd
never really understood why couples grieve so much about
miscarriage. Their baby hadn't even been born; maybe it was
nature's way of saying it shouldn't be. I figured babies are like
fruit on a tree — wind and rain don't knock off the good ones.

How easy it had been to be glib.

I put a protective hand on my belly. I was attached to this
baby, in more ways than one. Although Rob and I had been
married forever, this baby brought us closer, made us look to
the future, made me feel more committed.

We had already talked about what it might be like, look like.

We hoped it would have my eyesight and Rob's teeth, and we knew it was destined to have teenage acne. I had even indulged in a few giddy peeks into baby-clothing stores, children's bookstores, toy shops, and boutiques with window displays of pink desks and blue rocking horses.

We'd even talked names: Weston (Wes) for a boy, Ariel for a girl. My brother and sister-in-law hated the latter and swore they'd send no presents. Instead they sent an elaborately illustrated card that included a mock *New York Post* article entitled "First-Grader Shoots Parents Because of Name." The subhead read, "Jane-jane-bo-bane-banana-fana-fo-fane-me-mi-mo-mane Ackerman Taken into Custody by Juvenile Authorities. Legal Expert Says, 'No Jury on Earth Will Convict Her.' Horrified Aunt and Uncle Exclaim, 'We Warned Them.'" I'd put the card in my scrapbook after surveying their list of alternatives: Caliban, Daffodil, Mistletoe. Camembert, Pinecone, Snowflake. Toyota, Jubilation, Serendipity.

The point is this: I liked being small with child, with this child. We'd stopped thinking of it as some nameless, formless tadpole. Our baby-to-be had already become enormously important to us, had already put a lot of the flotsam and jetsam of our lives into perspective.

I was enjoying this early stage of pregnancy, pampering the baby and being pampered. Rob was cooking up lots of hearty meals ("Pregnancy Platters," he called them). I was taking prenatal vitamins, worrying about calcium instead of calories, and going from feeling starved to having no appetite. I also noticed, with some amusement, that I was prey to cravings. I was mad for potatoes, any shape, any style. Yet when Rob prepared an elegant dinner of fish and salad, I nearly cleaned my plate but, without realizing it, left a demure little pile of capers and pine nuts off to one side — an embarrassingly yuppie aversion.

Though often tired, I was happy to admit that I was having a smooth pregnancy. Yes, the taste of milk was getting old, and yes,

Chinese food looked unappetizingly brown, but I hadn't had morning sickness. All things considered, I was getting off easy.

I didn't want to start all over again. I wanted this pregnancy, this baby, this egg with this sperm, these parts of each of us that had joined together purposefully — miraculously — and were now one being waiting for birth.

My thoughts got darker.

If this baby doesn't make it, I wondered, how do I know I'll be able to carry another one to term?

At the doctor's office, Liz sat me down and took blood from the crook of my arm.

"We monitor this stuff carefully," she said. "Usually hormone levels increase steadily in the first trimester. When they don't, we like to check what's going on." She patted my arm. "Don't worry."

Easy for her to say. "I have just one question." My voice rose and cracked. "If this ovum is blighted, does that mean all my ova are blighted?"

"Don't worry," she repeated, handing me a tissue. I'd noticed that every room in their office had its own box of tissues. "All these tests and all this data get people so upset. They didn't used to have any of this."

I blew my nose and nodded. Our parents didn't argue about when to have a baby then fret week by week over that baby's development. They celebrated pregnancy with champagne and simply assumed all was well.

The drama quickly ended. Turned out my progesterone had caught up and everything was proceeding apace. Thank God. Nurse Liz also reassured me that I hadn't squashed, pickled, or poached my baby — but, she added, "Might as well stay away from ski slopes, bars, and hot tubs."

I felt like skipping home.

There had been nothing to fear but technology.

Lovemaking that night felt unusually close. Rob and I were both relieved, grateful, humbled. We were celebrating the health of our baby and — we'd just heard — the birth of our niece in Boston.

Sex in general those first weeks and that first trimester was, well, it depended on the night.

Springtime was making Rob extra lusty; pregnancy was making me extra drowsy. I tried to take catnaps — my old cat loved nothing more than for me to curl up beside her — but the phone would ring or I'd start worrying about deadlines or I'd think about all the calcium, protein, and leafy green vegetables I hadn't consumed that day, and next thing I knew, I'd be up making cream of chicken soup.

Sometimes I did sleep. But the fatigue of early pregnancy doesn't just go away. It's like low-grade mono. It's like suddenly finding that gravity's pull is a little stronger than it's ever been before. The lima bean inside me was small but growing fast and requiring lots of my energy to do so.

Occasionally I'd think, "I'll make a pot of coffee." But I'd read too many uncertain studies about caffeine, and whenever I'd have a cup, I wouldn't really enjoy it. If, while drinking, you're thinking, "Is this worth it?," it's not worth it. (Funny, though, how I never gave a thought to the caffeine in devil's food cake or chocolate-chip cookies. Even the tabloid headline "Sweet-Toothed Mom Delivers Chocolate-Covered Baby" didn't give me pause.)

By the time Rob came home from work each night and we'd had dinner and talked and gone through the mail and I'd read a chapter of some book and he'd watched the Yankees — sometimes through extra innings — it would be around eleven-thirty. He'd be ready for a bout in bed. I'd be about as frisky as an armchair.

26

Deep down, I also felt that, having successfully mated, Mother Nature now intended for me to be a mother hen: to sit quietly on my nest and behave myself.

The books I read said that such feelings, though passing, were normal. The books also reassured the mother-to-be that if her husband was suddenly turned off by her changing body, this too would pass.

That was not our problem.

Rob was turned on by my changing body. He found my fleeting new proportions arousing, and that further upset the temporary inequity of our lust. Truth is, my figure had never been better. My breasts were full and I still had my waist. What was not to like?

Except for one miserable year in junior high, I'd always been comfortable and content with my small breasts. But even I'll admit that I enjoyed feeling buxom, having a soupçon of cleavage, imagining that I was giving Dolly Parton a run for her money.

Mind you, to the untrained eye, it may have appeared that my body had changed not a whit.

But I was not to be disillusioned.

I'd step up to Robert, hoist my shirt above my neck, and say, "Can you believe how enormous I'm getting?" Or "Have you ever been married to someone so stacked?" Whereupon he would lunge at me, and I'd quickly pull back and say, "Gentle! They're tender!" or "I didn't say you could touch!" or "Honey, I'm exhausted."

Sex and the Pregnant Woman.

Poor Rob felt the gods were being mischievous, providing him with a wife with a Playmate of the Year body (okay, okay, I said I wasn't all that buxom) but sapping her of even her usual playfulness.

Not that I always said no. Sometimes I said yes, particularly if Rob kissed me provocatively *before* the first Yankee got to bat. Sex then would be more than fun. It would feel wonderful because, tired though I was, I was literally full of life, and that amazed and thrilled us. He'd pat my still-flat belly and marvel that it would grow enough to house our baby.

Rob also said I felt thicker and softer and confessed that it was kind of exciting, like making love to someone else without having to be unfaithful.

And of course being liberated from the rigmarole of diaphragms and goop made things more spontaneous.

So I tried to nap from time to time and Rob did all he could to keep me in the swing of things. He even bought cocoa butter and insisted on rubbing it on me to prevent stretch marks. I wasn't fooled. I knew he'd been wanting to do this for years. But for years, I'd been a killjoy — reluctant to soil the linens.

This time, his suggestion came the night before laundry day, and I didn't have the energy to put up any resistance. So I lay back, Rob rubbed, and, in a matter of minutes, I began to feel that I was turning into not Kafka's insect but a giant Almond Joy.

Cocoa butter wasn't the only thing Rob was bringing home. He arrived one day with a can of sardines (high in calcium), pregnancy tea (caffeine-free), Vitamin E oil (another stretch-mark preventative purchased for his rubbing pleasure), and bright pink tulips. He even bought me a Mother's Day gift at an antique store upstate: an old wooden high chair. The sentiment was sweet. But since I was only two and a half months pregnant, and since newborns can't sit up for six months or so, he was jumping the gun by over a year.

But that's what you do when you're expecting. You look ahead.

I, for instance, was obsessed about the future. I was eager to start showing. To put on billowy maternity dresses. To look conspicuously pregnant instead of looking the same — or worse, paunchy. My old clothes still fit all too well, and I was delighted when I found I had to wriggle into my jeans after taking them out of the dryer.

I also worried about the future. I worried that my baby would not be normal. I worried that my belly button would become an outie. I worried that I was not chugalugging enough milk. I worried that the letters on my computer screen were hazardous to my health. I worried that if my computer screen didn't get me, my microwave oven might. I worried about global warming, nuclear proliferation, overflowing landfills. About drug crimes in the city and deer ticks in the country. I worried that labor would hurt and that we'd soon discover that I had an embarrassingly low tolerance for pain.

As a kid, I had seen one too many westerns in which enormous ladies, stranded on the prairie, gave birth panting and screaming while husbands and neighbors mopped their brows with damp cloths.

In Sunday School, we'd read in the Bible that God's punishment to Eve for tempting Adam with the apple was pain in childbirth. Even then it had struck me as unfair that all woman-kind should suffer just because Eve had spunk.

More recently, I'd watched the *Today* show and heard Olympic runner Mary Decker Slaney say that even though she was in top condition, nothing had prepared her for the pain of labor.

Conception began to seem like just the first hurdle. Forceps, fetal monitors, twisted umbilical cords, emergency C-sections, pain, and fear: it seemed incredible that millions of healthy babies are born each year.

And then Oprah had to go and do an entire hour on child-birth. It was a beautiful afternoon in late May. I'd been at my word processor all day and was ready for a break. If I'd had a baby, I would have taken it out for a stroll. But I didn't have a baby. I had an inch-long embryo with little limbs and a tiny face. So I climbed in bed, propped up my feet, aimed the remote control at the T.V., and landed on *Oprah*. She'd rounded up three guest experts to enlighten us all about the experience of giving birth.

"I was in labor for fourteen hours," said one.

"I was in labor for eighteen hours," said the next.

"I was in pain for four solid days," said the third.

Maybe I should check out *Donahue*, I thought.

One of the guests allowed as to how birth is like trying to squeeze a brick out of your body.

"With the pain is there a sense of excitement that the baby is coming?" Oprah asked.

"No," said Guest Number Three without missing a beat. "For four days straight, I couldn't even open my mouth to breathe. All I could do was scream."

I wondered why the producers had chosen to send out a limo for this particular guest.

"I was so mean to my husband," she continued, "I was yelling, 'What have you done to me?'"

"You didn't think back on your night of passion?" Oprah asked.

"I cursed that night," said the guest. "I told my husband, 'Enjoy your son because that's it. I'm not having any more kids.'"

Hands shot up in the audience. One woman said she pushed so hard after her baby was born "that not only did my placenta come out, but my whole uterus came out."

I clutched my belly. I had not yet had morning sickness, but much more of this, and afternoon sickness would be a sure bet.

An ob/gyn pointed out that women have different pain thresholds and that second labors are often shorter. A Lamaze instructor said that labor is easier if you have taken classes and if you have a supportive person by your side.

After those reassuring insights and a commercial break, it was back to sensationalism. A guest said that when her water broke, she went to the hospital with a towel. "My tennis shoes were so sopped, they went squish squish squish against the floor."

Oprah's turn again: "Modesty is something you get over quickly if you're in labor," she said, "but one thing they don't tell you is that some women have a bowel movement right on the table."

Charming, I thought. A brand-new worry.

A caller phoned in. "Oprah, I love your show, but this is outrageous!"

Oprah seemed to realize that things had indeed gotten out of hand. "We don't want to do a disservice to those of you who are pregnant," she announced.

"Yo," I said aloud. "Too late." And then I made a deal with myself. I decided I'd try natural childbirth. Unless it hurt. And then I'd try drugs.

I'd let my husband knock me up. I might as well let my doctor knock me out.

I dreamed I bled in the toilet.

Though I worried a lot about my pregnancy during those first three months, it still seemed unreal. It even seemed odd that people always took my word for it when I said we were expecting. How did they know I wasn't making this up? Was I sure I wasn't? Was I sure all this napping wasn't just self-indulgence?

I told Dr. Romoff how tired I felt. "Hormones," he said. He thinks books on pregnancy overplay nausea and underplay fatigue. "You're in a haze because you're sedated by natural progesterone." He promised it would get easier.

He also told me to stop jogging.

"But I've been jogging since high school," I protested. "I have a great jogging partner. And the books all say you can keep doing what you've been doing."

"We're in the middle of a very hot, very muggy June, and it's just not worth it — the jostling or the exertion."

I wanted to argue. I wanted a second opinion. I wanted to whine, "It's not fair!" I didn't want to make sacrifices yet — there was plenty of time for that next year.

I'd miss meeting Patty for jogs around Riverside and Central Park. And now my thighs were going to chunk out along with the rest of me.

Then the Pollyanna in me looked at the bright side. My feet had been hurting lately anyway. Water retention? Weight gain? The heat wave? I often felt like putting them up not because I was tired, but because *they* were tired. Now I was under doctor's orders not to jog. Was that so bad? And if slowing down was good for the baby, what could be more important?

Dr. Romoff checked my weight, blood pressure, and abdomen and got out a doppler — a hand-held gizmo that magnifies sound and enables parents and physicians to hear the baby's heartbeat. He smeared something called Aquasonic Ultrasound Transmission gel on my belly. I was suddenly both excited and nervous.

He could tell I was hoping for a milestone and was quick with a disclaimer. "Don't worry if we can't hear it. You're only in your tenth week. It's still very early."

I lay back and he glided the doppler over the right side of my abdomen. There was sound everywhere: Gull-ump, Gull-ump, Gull-ump. I looked at him expectantly. "That's your pulse," he said.

He tried the middle of my abdomen: Gull-ump, Gull-ump, Gull-ump. I studied his expression. "Yours," he said.

He tried my left side, first up: Gull-ump, Gull-ump, Gull-ump. Then down: gullumpgullumpgullumpgullump.

"Bingo," he said. "That's your baby."

My baby. My baby! I smiled at the ceiling. And I listened to my baby's speedy little heart, beating sure, beating strong, filling the room, proving aloud that it was for real, that everything was all right, that it was alivealivealivealive.

The haze finally lifted. And just in time. My book was coming due and I was tired of dozing off, leaning onto the keyboard of my word processor, then snapping awake to see a string of *llllll*'s or *ssssss*'s where I'd just been making careful edits.

I'd worked at home for years but had never before been so aware of how close my office was to my bed. Sure, I'd been tempted at times by the nearby refrigerator. But never by my bed, my beckoning bed, my downy soft bed, my right-around-the-corner bed, my all-I'd-have-to-do-is-kick-off-my-shoes-and-hop-in bed. . . .

Everyone had promised that my energy would come back in the second trimester, and thank heavens it did. But when the ob/gyn pointed out that since Rob and I both have some Eastern European Jewish ancestry, one of us should be tested to see if we were carriers of a rare but fatal disease, I didn't think twice: I chose Rob for the job.

"I've given enough blood already," I said when he returned from work.

"Tay-Sachs? I've never even heard of Tay-Sachs. Why should I get tested for something I've never heard of?"

"Because Dr. Yale said to."

"Well, that's ridiculous! She's crazy."

No one, not even my husband, slanders my ob/gyn and gets away with it. Mock my dentist. Malign my stockbroker. Criticize my hairstylist. But lay off my family and my ob/gyns. I'd placed the care of my unborn child in Drs. Yale and Romoff's hands, and they were above reproach.

"I'm getting needles stuck in me left and right," I said. "It's your turn." I kissed him and added, "Wimp."

Rob was silent.

"Remember that nice dream you told me about?" I asked. "The one where someone handed you a baby and within weeks you'd taught it to walk and talk? Things aren't that smooth."

34

He imagined the road ahead as Easy Street; I saw it paved with boulders. He thought Life with Baby would be a breeze; I envisioned tornadoes.

"Okay, okay," Rob said. He made the appointment, crossed town, and gave blood. Blood, which, weeks later, was given the doctor's thumbs-up.

The test we decided *not* to take was amniocentesis. I'd started noticing Down's syndrome babies and handicapped kids as much as the next pregnant lady, but my doctors assured me that, since I was just thirty, "There's no reason to take the test."

The odds of having a Down's syndrome baby go up with a woman's age, they said, but statistics were still on my side. The slight risk of Down's didn't warrant running the slight risk of losing the baby because of the procedure. Less than one percent of women have miscarriages as a result of amnio, they said, but nonetheless, at my age I could skip it.

I didn't argue. I wasn't pushing for more expenses or discomfort. And Rob and I had already decided that even if I had amnio, we wouldn't ask to find out the baby's sex. For us, it would have felt like opening our Christmas present on the Fourth of July. I feared it might make the baby's arrival anticlimactic. In the delivery room, when my doctor said, "It's a ———!" I didn't want to think, "I know." I wanted to think, "A ———!!! How wonderful!"

A friend had recently told us about his wife's disconcerting sonogram. "First the technician said we were going to have a girl, and I started picturing little dresses, and I was all excited. Then he said, 'No, no, my mistake. You're going to have a boy,' and I was happy, but I was also sad that this lovely girl we'd just been given was being taken away. So fine, I'm studying the sonogram and picturing a boy — roughhousing, ball games, father-son talks. I think I can even make out his little hand waving to me. Then suddenly the technician says, 'You know, it's still so early, I'm afraid I can't be certain what the sex is.' It was horrible. I felt like I'd been given a daughter and a son, and they were both spirited away, and I was sent home empty-handed."

Many couples love learning the sex of their future child. But when people asked me, "Do you know if it's a boy or a girl?" (the modern-day follow-up to "When are you due?"), I took an odd pride in my old-fashioned ignorance, in shaking my head and saying, "Nope."

It would have been practical to know if we should paint the nursery blue or pink, if we should invest in sailor suits or party dresses, if we needed to settle on a boy's name or a girl's name. But we liked the mystery.

We were eager to welcome our baby, male or female, and we considered the suspense part of the fun.

I delivered my book the day it was due. Was a book like a baby? You produce it, shape it, work on it, but ultimately have to let it go, wish it well, and hope it gets accepted in the world. Maybe. Yet you have more control over a book than over a child, I realized, with some trepidation.

I walked home to the Upper West Side from the publisher's office midtown and thought about new projects. As a freelance writer, I'm my own boss. The problem: I can be a slave driver. My mother raised me to work hard, to think in terms of goals and accomplishments, to have something to show for myself at the end of each day. I tend to push, push, push.

But in a little over five months, I'd be push, push, pushing in the maternity ward. And so I did a remarkable thing: I decided to give myself a break. I decided to take a chill pill along with my prenatal vitamin.

Some pregnant women work harder than ever during pregnancy, thinking, "If not now, when?" I was wondering about taking it easier, thinking, "If not now, when?"

Could we afford it? Yes, if my sabbatical were brief. When Rob and I first got married, my annual income was greater than his. I even wrote an article for *Bride's* titled "When You're Earning and He's Learning" about our struggle when he was in grad school. Now the tables were turning, he had a dependable income, and I felt I could take a little downtime. Besides, I had just handed in a 336-page manuscript.

Whether you have a job or not, one of the happy side effects of pregnancy is that because you are making a baby, you feel productive even when you're being lazy. Lately when I watched late-night T.V., instead of also reading a magazine, doing my scrapbook, or organizing my sock drawer, I'd just pat my busy belly and feel content. If I felt energetic, I might get out a bag of microwave popcorn and nuke a snack. It may have appeared that I was just another couch potato, but look again: I was a model of productivity.

What a liberating feeling! The Puritan ethic is strong, but for once my body had the upper hand. Summer was here and I was actually thinking about relaxing and enjoying it. About hanging out, barefoot and pregnant.

Maybe there is a hidden advantage in having a baby in your thirties — you've made a few strides and can consider taking a career break.

I decided to visit my grandfather in Texas.

I chose an aisle seat on the flight down (I knew I'd be making repeated trips to the lavatory), then took a van to the house where my mother grew up.

"Why, you're not showing a bit," my stepgrandmother, Morine, said, probably by way of a compliment. She seemed disappointed and I was, too. I was four months along. I *wanted* to be showing. It was frustrating that even in my roomy maternity top and stretch pants, it still looked like I was pulling a fast one. When would I stop feeling like a sausage in my old clothes, an imposter in my new ones?

Granddad and I greeted each other with "Howdy Pahdner" and a hug, as we'd been doing since I was a girl. He suggested I get settled in the guest room. I remembered my parents' last trip together to Texas and thought, but did not say, "You mean the room where Dad died?" Life, death, life. My grandmother died here eleven years ago. My father, five. If Granddad was at peace with the memories, I didn't want to cause a fuss.

He offered to help carry my bags upstairs. But though I was pregnant, he was ninety, so I casually insisted on doing it myself.

We ate a late lunch of ham, black-eyed peas, salad, watermelon pickles, corn muffins, and blackberry cobbler. Granddad had been a doctor for fifty-five years, so I brought up the subject of delivering babies.

Morine interjected, "Every time we go out, someone says, 'Dr. Little, you delivered me.' And these people are sometimes fifty, sixty years old!" She said lots of babies were named for him. "The parents would be having trouble getting pregnant, and your granddad would give them some advice, and next thing you know, they'd be having a son and naming him Aubrey."

"What'd you tell them, Granddad?"

"Well, it depended. Sometimes I'd tell the women to douche with baking soda instead of vinegar, which is too acidic, and I'd tell the men to wear boxers instead of briefs, and that would be enough. But if I thought they needed to hear more," he paused and grinned, "I might tell them to sleep with a sack of potatoes under their bed."

I loved my granddad's mix of medical science and folk remedies. Whenever I phoned with an ache or pain, he was as likely to tell me, for instance, to eat more bananas (for potassium) as he was to recommend medicine. I also loved his stories about getting paid during the Depression. Patients who couldn't offer money offered eggs, chickens, pies, portraits, and sometimes a quilt.

"Do you remember the first time you delivered a baby?"

"Heck, I delivered thirty babies before I was out of med school. Most times I went to people's homes."

"Were you scared at first?"

"Scared? No." He sipped his buttermilk.

"Weren't you scared but pretending to be brave?"

"No, I wasn't scared. It comes naturally. And I was damned good at home deliveries. I used to teach students how to do it. I enjoyed delivering babies. I always felt I was accomplishing something."

"Did you ever deliver any deformed babies, or have real trouble getting a baby out?" I locked my hands over my stomach as I asked him the questions I was afraid to ask my ob/gyns.

Granddad took a deep breath. "I got 'em all out. Sometimes

their heads looked like sweet potatoes, but that lasted only a few days. Listen, I remember being apprehensive when your grandmother was pregnant. But look how many healthy babies there are out there. Don't you go worrying about that."

"I haven't felt any kicking yet, but I shouldn't worry about that either, right?

"No, you shouldn't." He said things were much safer nowadays. "Used to be, some doctors scarcely knew to keep their hands clean. But it's hard for doctors today, too. If a baby arrives with six toes, the obstetrician gets sued."

"Granddad, you know how doctors tell women not to drink or smoke during pregnancy? Is it true they never did that way back when?"

"They didn't have to. Most women didn't drink or smoke."

He pushed back his plate and said he was going upstairs to take a nap.

Bedtime for all of us was nine o'clock — after dinner, *Jeopardy,* and the news. I wasn't particularly tired as I lay, pregnant, on my father's deathbed.

I thought about Dad's last words: "Anybody want to go to a movie?" No one did, so he had turned in early. A movie. I liked knowing he felt that good when he went to bed for the last time.

For me, the phone call came midmorning. "Dad died in his sleep," my brother Mark said. I remember calling an airline, being put on hold, hearing an endless Muzak version of "Raindrops Keep Falling on My Head."

When I got to Texas, Mom explained, crying, that her sister had arrived, and that she and Aunt Norah had stayed up late talking and had gone to sleep in their old twin beds. Mom wasn't with Dad when he died, and in the morning, she'd gone in and out of their room several times but had assumed he was sleeping late.

At nine-thirty, she'd nudged him. He was cold.

She'd screamed. Granddad appeared, but it didn't take a degree in medicine to tell that Dad was dead.

The autopsy revealed that it was a massive heart attack. I liked knowing it was massive, that nothing could have been done.

I also felt that Dad, then sixty-eight, might have chosen such an exit — "before a petal fell," as one friend put it.

But his quick peaceful death left the rest of us stranded, reeling, bereft.

That night, in that room, I had a nightmare. I dreamed my family was driving through a woods when suddenly our car stopped. "Let's keep going!" I said. "I'm spooked." But Mom said Dad had to rest. "Let's put Dad in the back and you drive," I said, but Dad had already gotten out. I went to look for him and heard him reciting a Shakespearean farewell. I hugged Dad tight and said, "NO! You can't leave! I love you so much and so does Eric and so does Mark!" He said he'd been thinking about the children. I was sobbing and Mom put her arm around me and said we had to keep going but that Dad couldn't go anymore.

I woke up, wet with tears, and I thought I would never ever be able to handle my father's death.

But then, turning my head on the pillow, opening my eyes to the Texas sunlight, I realized I had "handled" it: Dad was dead and I had survived.

Over orange juice, Granddad said he dreamed I had a baby girl and that we came to visit. I didn't share my dream.

That afternoon we drove to the falls of Wichita Falls, recently honored by a visit from the *Today* show's Willard Scott. I remembered one of my first drives with Granddad. I'd sat in the backseat, discovered his black medical bag, and had a grand time rearranging pills and sticking Band-Aids all over myself.

This time I sat up front as we pulled into Crestview Cemetery. I helped Granddad out of the car and our shadows stretched long on the grass and clover above my father and grandmother and greatgrandparents. We held hands silently. Before we left, Granddad offered his first wife a bouquet, and I tucked daisies in the vase by the block letters of my father's name, my name.

Driving back, we stopped at a take-out place to pick up fried chicken. A man in his late fifties approached us. "Dr. Little," he said. "Brandon Pierce. You delivered me."

I beamed.

"This here is my granddaughter," Granddad said. "She's expecting in December."

"Well, you must be mighty proud."

Granddad clasped his hand on my shoulder. He did take pride in his family's accomplishments — diplomas, promotions, books. But I knew nothing pleased him more than to know that his only granddaughter was pregnant, that his blood was coursing on. "As long as you kids have kids of your own," he had told me at breakfast, "I know I will never die."

Rob helped me in with my bags. "How are you?" I asked. "And how's Chanda?"

Chanda was our seventeen-year-old chocolate-point Siamese. My family brought her home when I was an eighth-grader and she was a kitten. Rob had been warned that we were a package deal, and Dad could hardly wait to hand the cat over when we got married.

Chanda moved with Rob and me to Columbus, Ohio; Evanston, Illinois; and finally Manhattan. Rob didn't mind sharing our bed with her year after year, and she, now old, didn't mind ending up an apartment cat.

During the day, she slept and purred in the blocks of sunlight that moved across our living room. At night, she yowled. Often at 3:00 A.M. Rob usually slept through her antics, while I would stumble to the kitchen to sprinkle some water on her food and give it a stir. Poor cat could hardly see or smell anymore and needed to be reminded that her bowl was not empty.

I didn't enjoy getting up before sunrise. But I figured it was good training for motherhood. And you can't teach an old cat new tricks. Besides, taking care of her was my job.

Then my ob/gyns tested my blood, and found that despite the dozens of cats that had padded in and out of my life, I was not immune to toxoplasmosis. They spoke to me gravely about infection from feline feces and said — in short — to stay away from cat poop.

"You're kidding!" Rob had said when he first heard about it.

"Disgusting!" he said later, when, resigned, he sifted through the sand of Chanda's litter box.

"Rob, I hope you were nice to her while I was in Texas," I said, as I put down my purse, kicked off my shoes, and lifted her bony purring body to my chest. Pitiful cat was losing weight at about the pace I was gaining.

I called my mother to tell her how well her father was. She and my stepfather, Lewis, had just gone to Cape Cod for the summer, a tradition his family had enjoyed for years.

"And how are *you* feeling, pumpkin?"

Pumpkin. Would I call my kid pumpkin when he or she was thirty?

"Fine." I thanked her for reading and editing my book and told her I'd handed it in. "The baby still hasn't kicked, and I'm getting occasional headaches and middle-of-the-night charley horses. But I can't complain. I'm not a June balloon."

"I remember having leg cramps when I was pregnant. You know how to flex your feet and pull your lip to stop them?"

"Yeah. It's not that big a deal, just a rude awakening." I liked it when my mother shared a memory from her pregnancy. She had worked until the week before each of us was born and usually claimed that she sort of missed out on the pregnancy experience.

"How's Robert?"

"Fine. Everyone's calling him 'Stud' and he's eating it up. On Father's Day we went to an ice-cream store that offered free mini-sundaes to dads, and I asked if he could have one since he's a father-to-be. That was his first official perk."

I added that he's been baseball-crazed lately and that he'd gone on about some big game on T.V. last night. "Did Lewis watch it?"

"No. We had lobster for dinner and walked out on the pier to see the full moon. Then we came home and went to bed."

"Sounds nice," I said.

"It is. Sublime."

My mother, a grandmother? I still couldn't see it.

I know I've gone on and on about the enormity of my breasts, and I know I should stop, but the most amazing thing about pregnancy is how your body keeps changing. My body hadn't changed — really changed — since puberty. My breasts hadn't grown since tenth grade. I had scarcely worn a bra in fifteen years.

It was time to go shopping. Only this time I'd be going alone, without my mother waiting discreetly outside the dressing room to whisper well-chosen words of encouragement.

I went to Mothercare, which specializes in baby and maternity wear. The clerk inadvertently offended me with the old "Gee, you're hardly showing" line. I went to the Town Shop, which specializes in lingerie. There the saleswoman showed proper respect for my burgeoning bust. "Oh, yes, you should definitely be wearing a support bra," she said. To my delight, she even scolded me for not coming in earlier.

I ducked into the dressing room, tried on several bras, and chose two. Then I noticed their size, 36C.

36C! No! Last I'd checked, I was a 32AA. Surely I hadn't skipped the A's and B's. This must be like when you try on a designer dress and the tag says size 3, but you know it's just flattery. I looked again: Vanity Fair 36C.

A C! On me! I blushed with triumph and resolved to save a tag for evidence for my scrapbook. I couldn't wait to tell Rob, Jen, Patty, my mother.

Strange, but during this period, I lost all modesty about my body. I almost felt that it wasn't my body, my petite particular body. It was a generic pregnant woman's body, a case study, a textbook example of the changes incurred during gestation. I even flashed for interested girlfriends so they could see my growing belly and the network of blue lines crisscrossing my breasts. The effect reminded me of the transparent models we studied in biology when we learned about veins and arteries.

My body had become a curiosity and I didn't mind. Many pregnant women object when strangers touch their bellies, but I thought I might find it endearing when someone I'd never met acknowledged my future son or daughter with an affectionate pat. People are entitled to welcome in the next generation, aren't they? I practically considered my own pregnancy public domain.

And now, a 36C! I laughed as I paid for my bras. I imagined I was in a musical in which the ring of the cash register was the first note of an elaborate melody of drum rolls, trumpets, and violins. I could see myself skipping out the door and bursting into song:

> I feel busty, oh, so busty,
> I feel busty, and lusty — hooray!
> Oh, I'm glowing
> Cuz I'm showing —
> I finally look pregnant today!

I just hoped I could appreciate being flat again when this was all over.

I can't believe my wife is a mammal," Rob was saying to Miguel as they smeared themselves with sunscreen. "I mean, she's got this baby inside her who is going to come out and suckle on her for months and months before it can walk around."

I dried my hair and spread my towel on the sand. "I prefer to think of myself as one of those Russian *matryoshka* dolls," I said. "You know, inside the first is another then another then another." Generations of *babushkas*.

Beth, Ed, and Susan came out of the water. "Do you believe my arm?" I showed them where my veins had been assaulted the week before. "A spina bifida test. The nurse missed and now I look like an I.V. drug user."

"You look great," Susan protested. "Pregnancy agrees with you. Hasn't everyone been saying that?"

"Just my mom. And she hasn't seen me for a month."

We were enjoying this late-summer day at Jones Beach: the sun, waves, picnic, company. But we were each aware of an unspoken awkwardness, too. I was beginning to fill out my maternity suit while Beth and Susan looked lithe and sexy in their bikinis. I looked wistfully at their flat bellies; they looked wistfully at my distended one.

Beth was quiet but seemed grumpy. Ed said it was "that time of the month" — a double curse in their case.

Susan talked about her miscarriage and said it was frustrating that she hadn't gotten pregnant again. I remembered her birthday celebration weeks earlier. Miguel had served champagne and I'd asked for "just a drop," feeling self-conscious and guilty that even on her birthday, I was a reminder of the wish that still eluded her.

I got up. God it was hot. It had been sticky all summer and I felt thankful that I wasn't in full bloom.

47

Susan and I walked to the edge of the water and sat down. "So how's sex?" she asked.

I laughed. "I'm more into it than I was the first trimester." "And Rob?"

"Rob's always into it. He wants to jump my bones even when they're hard to find." I adjusted my sunglasses. "His sister just leant me a Jane Fonda tape and some maternity clothes. The clothes are wonderful, but I can't bring myself to put on the tape."

"If I get pregnant," Susan said, "maybe we'll join a prenatal exercise class together." The beach was full of toddlers, each accompanied by pails and shovels and parents. Their oiled nearly naked bodies shone in the sun, and some shrieked with primal joy. "Are these kids cute or what?"

"Adorable," I said. One little girl, her tummy protruding, waddled over to us and offered Susan a handful of wet sand.

"Thank you," she said, accepting it graciously.

The girl walked away. "Did you notice that she and I have the exact same profile?" I asked.

"No," Susan replied. "I'm far too polite."

On the car ride back, Rob announced that we were going to start looking for a bigger apartment in Manhattan. The idea of moving made us nervous and giddy, and I knew it signaled the end of my laid-back summer.

For months off and on, both Beth and Ed and Susan and Miguel had been making noises about leaving New York — moving someplace cleaner, cheaper, quieter, more civil. We kept hoping that they were here to stay, that they were just feeling a restlessness that would disappear upon conception, if not sooner.

For us, conception is what prompted our decision to look around. Like many expectant couples, we realized we had to take action before we outgrew our home.

It had finally dawned on us that I wasn't just pregnant — we were *going to have a baby.* A baby who would need room to grow.

Government warning: According to the surgeon general, women should not drink alcoholic beverages during pregnancy because of the risk of birth defects.

Now that I was virtually teetotaling, I was constantly amazed at how much everyone else drank. Now that I was eating relatively nutritiously, I was astounded at how much junk food everyone else ate.

"Well don't get holier-than-thou about it," Rob warned.

"I'm trying not to."

We both had to fight the urge to proselytize to other couples in their thirties. Even I, recent convert, was tempted to tell married friends that they shouldn't wait forever before trying to start a family. "You'll never really feel ready. There's never really a good time," I'd sometimes say, amazed at how quickly I'd begun to sound like Rob. "You don't want to miss the boat," I'd want to add. Fortunately I still recognized reproduction as a loaded topic and tended to broach it gingerly or not at all.

Besides, for us the test was still ahead as to whether we'd been irretrievably foolhardy or wonderfully wise.

Pregnancy was turning out to be a pleasant surprise, but for me, pregnancy — even the relatively easy second trimester — had its drawbacks. They say mothers are self-sacrificing, guilt-ridden worrywarts. Yet I hadn't expected all that to begin *before* birth.

I was supposed to go to England in November to help spread the word about the British publication of my first book, *Girltalk.* But since I'd be eight months along by then, I called to cancel the trip: my first professional stepping-aside in the name of motherhood, and I hated to do it.

Sacrifice, sacrifice.

A woman in my building told me that when she was pregnant she started every day with a glass of juice, a glass of milk, a scrambled egg, a piece of toast, and a fresh fruit salad topped with yogurt. Me? I just poured myself some cereal (and maybe a café au lait, mostly *lait*) then grazed all day long. Was that good enough? Should I be dining on high-calcium collards and kale, oysters and figs?

Guilt, guilt.

And why wasn't my kid kicking? How come I still had to say no when the ob/gyn asked if I'd "detected any movement"?

Worry, worry.

A new-mother friend called from California.

"How are you feeling?" she asked. "Oh, wait, the baby just spit up — hang on."

I hung on.

"I'm in the middle of breast-feeding. It's so great, having a baby. You're going to love it. He's so cute. I've got to send you a picture — if I can ever get dressed and over to the camera shop! I'm telling you, getting out of the house is a Major Challenge. Oh, and we're teething, which is a bitch. But he is so precious, his itty-bitty fingers and button toes. He's got his eyes closed right now and is sucking so peacefully. Oh, damn, he just puked. Listen, I'll have to call you back."

What had Rob and I done?

I know, I know, when it's *your* baby — *your* baby's button toes, *your* baby's spit-up — it's supposed to be magic. But is it really?

Despite moments of doubt, Rob and I were caught up in the anticipation. When I found out that he was going to meet Dr. Spock, I was beside myself with excitement.

Rob does special effects and props for films and T.V. commercials. He can make walnuts dance for a chocolate-bar ad or have hamburgers tuck themselves into buns for a fast food spot. When milk has to splash onto a bowl of cornflakes, he stirs in Elmer's glue to get just the right consistency. When it has to rain on film, he's sometimes the guy offstage with water trucks, fire hoses, and sprinkler heads. It's complicated kid stuff and Rob loves playing Mr. Wizard.

Like me, he's free-lance. But he doesn't work alone; he works on set for different production companies. His hours are long and unpredictable — except when the phone doesn't ring and he has an unexpected free day (or worrisome week) off. Every once in a while, he works with someone famous: Bob Hope, Christie Brinkley, Jane Pauley, Latoya Jackson. This time he would be working behind the scenes on a shoot in which Spock would talk about everything from babies to Vietnam.

Spock! Not the Vulcan. The doctor! I couldn't believe it. I collect autographed books and begged Rob to get him to do a personal signing.

"You'll have to pick up a copy of *Dr. Spock's Baby and Child Care*," I said.

"We already have a copy."

"We have it in paperback. We need it in hardback."

Rob looked puzzled.

"Pleeeease," I pleaded.

He said he'd see what he could do.

And that night he came home with one of the best gifts he's ever given me: a $19.95 edition of the baby doctor's classic, penned with these perfect words:

"To Carol, with envy and love —   Ben Spock"

Women and children first," I said, "and right now I'm both." I helped myself to some of Lewis's bouillabaisse at his buffet table in Provincetown.

"You're so smug," he said with affection.

"I know I am. It's terrible. We're just excited."

"Marybeth is too. Last week she started to lactate."

"Oh, Lewis!" Mom said, frowning, beaming.

My mother the Southern belle had done it again: married a witty New York journalist who not only loved to cook, but loved to make off-color remarks to which she could feign offense. Lewis had been Mom's boss at the *New York Times Sunday Magazine* thirty years earlier when he was a hotshot editor, she, a go-getter writer, and both had families to go home to. When Mom changed jobs, they lost touch. For decades. Then Dad died. Then Lewis's wife died. Mom and Lewis had mutual friends and she dropped him a sympathy note. He called some time afterward and, after a summer of letters and phone calls, the sparks were flying. Now they were married and palpably in love; each clearly felt lucky to have found another *grand amour*.

When I had first met Lewis, I extended my hand, but, to my embarrassment, my eyes filled with tears. It took me several minutes to regain my composure, yet only several more to see what my mother saw in him: a quick mind, a sexy smile, a generous spirit. Qualities my Dad had had as well. They say it's the happily married widows and widowers who are most eager to marry again, and I didn't begrudge Mom this radiant new chapter of her life.

I stirred the bouillabaisse. Rob and I had spent the last seven hours driving and had eaten only carrots, grapes, and sandwiches. I was hungry.

"Have I shown you my *linea nigra?*" Lewis teased as he lifted his T-shirt to his navel.

"Lewis, put your shirt down," my mother scolded, shaking her head.

"I don't have one," I said. "Gigantic bosoms and a prominent stomach, but no dark line." I stood and pulled my top up a few inches.

"Would everybody please sit down and keep their clothes on?" Mom asked. We all took a seat and held hands before dinner — my mother's silent way of saying grace.

After the dishes, Mom and I lay down on the bed in a guest room. Rob and Lewis were watching a Yankees game. Outside it was gray and thundering.

"So what's the next book? *Babytalk?*"

"Maybe. That's what everyone keeps asking."

I told her about the photo shoot for the cover of *Girltalk About Guys*. "They used five Ford models, all teens and preteens. Some were gorgeous, but some were just sort of wholesome." I remembered my friends' and my wishing we could be models when we were in high school. The magazines made it seem so glamorous. "Think little one here will be able to earn top dollar just for smiling?" I gave my belly a pat. "Course it depends in part on whether it ever grows any legs. By now it's supposed to have eyebrows and fingernails, and it still hasn't even kicked."

My mother started to answer but I interrupted with a whisper. "Wait. Put your hand right here."

It wasn't a kick I was feeling. It was a shifting of weight. A tight hardness where my belly is usually soft.

"Feel anything?" I asked.

Mom was quiet. She moved her palm to another spot.

Then I definitely felt it: a wave rippling inside me, a body in my body, a stirring, nudging, tapping from within. Knock, knock. Who's there?

"I felt that," my mother exclaimed. She spread her fingers over the spot.

The quickening, at long last. I'd been so cautious. It was thrilling to be sure.

In high school, I'd asked my brother Mark how you'd know if you had an orgasm. "If you had one, you'd know," he'd said. But this baby business was subtle. They say second-time-around mothers recognize fetal movement early, but until now, I was scared to give myself permission to acknowledge the rumblings for what they were.

Mom said it brought back memories of when she had felt each of us inside her, like a floating astronaut attached by the umbilical cord. She said she was honored my baby had waited until now to make its move.

"Pretty neat mother-daughter moment," I agreed.

Rob walked in. "Feel right here," I said.

"My God!" he said after a pause. "There's something alive inside my wife!"

When we got back to New York, I left a message on Seth's answering machine congratulating him on finishing his medical exams and telling him that the baby had finally kicked. I signed off "Buxomly yours, Carol."

He left a reply on our machine: "As soon as I walked out of the exam I dialed my machine and heard your message. I am indeed pleased to be a member of the leisure class again. I'm even happier that the woman with cleavage is going to have a baby with legs. How very very exciting."

It was. It was.

Even my shadow is pregnant, I noticed one Saturday. I was nearing the end of my second trimester. My stomach was big and hard and lopsided, and strangers always looked at it before meeting my eyes. Like when you wear a T-shirt with words emblazoned across the front, and passersby stare at your chest before looking up.

When I got back from the ob/gyn's, Rob was on the phone with his sister Lisa.

"She's fine," he was saying. "Bigger."

I got on. "I'm big as a house."

"Well, maybe a Winnebago," he said.

I imagined that sideways I looked like the child's picture in *The Little Prince*. The one of a boa eating an elephant — the one grown-ups all think is a hat.

Sarah, our new niece, began to wail in the background.

"So Lisa, would you say motherhood is everything it's cracked up to be?" Rob asked.

"And then some," she answered. "Listen, I'll call you back."

I joined Rob in the bedroom and started undressing.

"I thought your appointment was at three. What took you so long?"

"Dr. Romoff had to rush off to deliver a baby, and Dr. Yale's schedule was already full."

Rob studied me. Even he was transfixed by my belly. "You really are huge."

"You ain't seen nothin' yet."

"No, you got giant. When did this happen?"

"Mid-March," I said dryly. "You were there." But I knew what he meant. Some days it seemed I was growing by the hour. When I saw gargantuan women in the street or at the ob/gyn's, I'd think, is my belly going to do that? *Can* my belly do that?

True, when Rob and I went out, I usually felt cute, albeit dumplinglike, in my borrowed maternity clothes. And I enjoyed the extra attention a pregnant woman gets. At parties there was never a dearth of small talk. I'd be having my own private feeding frenzy at the hors d'oeuvre table when somebody would say, "Congratulations! What month are you in?" and all ice would be broken.

But despite my hurry to start showing, part of me now missed being slim. When I tried to squeeze through a narrow space, I'd get stuck. When I tried to slip by something, I'd knock into it instead. One night I dreamed I fit into my jeans. I was delighted and couldn't believe I'd been living in sweats and maternity outfits when I had jeans — jeans! — to wear.

"According to Dr. Yale," I informed Rob, "I'm carrying small." Of course, every pound counts on a five-two frame. "She says she can't pinch an inch, that it's 'all baby, no fat.'" I liked that: all baby, no fat. It sounded like a T.V. commercial.

I'd started feeling tired again, yet napping had become next to impossible. Our apartment was now listed with every realtor in town and our phone rang off the hook. I had to keep the place not just tidy, but spic-and-span. Worse, I had to be friendly to all the people who came snooping into our halls, rooms, and closets, then made quick getaways, clearly underwhelmed.

We'd put a lot of work into our apartment and the realtors' listings made us proud. One read: "Brilliant S/W light floods this pretty-as-a-picture hi-ceil move-in cond co-op with lovely redone kitchen, large square LR, corner MBR with 4 windows, utterly charming views of gardens, brownstone rooftops & sky. Loc in magnif 24 hr attended prewar in fine W. 80s." Others came under the headlines "New, Mint and Near Park," "Sunfilled Find," "Indian Summer," and finally, "Owner Must Sell."

Traffic we had. Prospective buyers arrived by the dozen, each as hopeful as we were. But we could always see it on their faces: our layout was awkward, our rooms small, our kitchen tiny, our view overrated.

"How many square feet do you have?" they'd ask.

"I'm not sure," I'd answer, afraid to say, "Under nine hundred."

Then the previous week, a redheaded lawyer and his fiancée looked at our home not once but twice and scheduled a Tuesday-night appointment at 7:45 for her parents to come by.

This was it.

At 7:30 the place was shining and ready for white-glove inspection. It was a hot night, so I put the air conditioner on full blast for a moment or two.

Big mistake. At 7:40 when I did a final check, I found I had a blackout in the living room.

The fuse box. I had an inkling where it was, but where were the fuses? I turned off the air conditioner, grabbed the cordless phone, dialed Rob at work, and frantically started lighting decorative candles. In our household, any fuse-related task was considered a Rob-job. Why, oh why had I let myself become a helpless female?

"May I speak to Robert, please?"

"He's on set."

Say it isn't so. Actors, directors, best boys, gaffers, grips, stylists, prop men, production assistants, the camera crew, and my husband all hard at work. Do Not Disturb. I screwed up my courage. "It's sort of an emergency. It'll take only two seconds."

A long pause at the other end. "Hang on."

"Rob, I'm sorry. Where do we keep fuses, and which fuse turns on the living-room light?"

"This is an emergency?"

"Our buyers are probably in the elevator on the way up."

"Oh, Jesus."

"Just tell me."

"In the middle drawer of the dresser, in the back. I don't know if they're all good. Some might be old."

"Great. Okay, thanks. Cross your fingers."

I began experimenting. I sprinted to the living room to see if it was still dark. It was. Only now, so was the bedroom. I dashed back and forth, cursing and replacing fuses wildly, when suddenly footsteps boomed in the hall. The doorbell rang. "Let there be light," I said as, hand on knob, I stretched to see if I'd finally hit on the right combination. Yes! The apartment was awash in light. I thought, Thank you, God. I owe you one.

But it was not to be. Red flags waved everywhere: the candles glowed; the fuse box hung open; I was a nervous wreck. I confessed all, stammering foolishly that it was a first, that I'd never before had the opportunity to change a fuse.

"I take it the apartment needs rewiring?" The father asked.

The realtor phoned the next day. "The lawyer called. He said they aren't ready to make a bid after all."

Who could blame them? Ah well, there was still that German pediatrician who'd come once alone and once with his mother, but who hadn't made an offer. Maybe he'd come back. Selling to a pediatrician would be better for our karma anyway.

"So are we still mad at each other?" Rob asked.

"You tell me," I said as I stretched in bed.

Our wires had been crossing lately. *Our* fuses had grown short. Rob had been working late night after night and this moving stuff was stressing me out.

The day before, a realtor had shut the door of my office closet, which is where we keep Chanda's litter box. I was out and the poor cat finally relieved herself in a box full of papers — my only copy, it turned out, of the book I'd just handed in.

Then that morning Rob locked me out. I'd already been miffed at him. He'd neglected to give me an important phone message. He'd thrown out the newspaper before I'd read it. And he'd lunged ahead and told his father that we were considering using his name as a middle name. ("Unfair," I said. "I could tell my grandfather the same thing.")

Now I'd asked Rob to get milk (he'd promised to bring some

home after work), and he said he didn't feel like going out. "Fine," I'd said curtly. "I'll go get some. But I can't find my key, so don't leave."

When I returned, Rob was in the shower, oblivious to my ringing, knocking, kicking, and pounding.

"You didn't have to get hysterical," he said, when at last he let me in.

I sniffed. "It's my pregnancy and I can cry if I want to."

"It goes with the territory?"

"I'm entitled."

But why was I so on edge? Hormones? Fatigue? Fear of the changes up ahead?

Or is it that when you're pregnant, you begin to feel dependent and vulnerable, no matter how modern and strong your marriage? Perhaps I was experiencing some deep-seated fear of abandonment. When you're pregnant, you want your husband to be extra loving. A no-big-deal tiff feels like a big deal. Dime-a-dozen spats hurt a dozen times more.

"I don't want us to stay mad," Rob said.

"Okay. Then let's call a cease-fire. Life is too short."

"You're too short," he replied.

"And you're a jerk-face," I said, always glad to have the last word.

Hemlines were heading north and since my legs were one of the few parts of me that wasn't swollen, I decided to get in on the action. Lisa had lent me a dress with a waistline that could be moved up, so I took a breath, hiked it high, and consulted the mirror. I was pretty sure I looked ridiculous, but I figured, this is New York. In New York, it's hard to look ridiculous.

I put on new panty hose and went out to pick up a copy of *Modern Bride*. I had an article in it called, "Keep Your Marriage a Ten" — ironic considering our marital mood the previous weekend.

Turned out that was only half the irony. Did the newsstand salesman smirk because I was the picture of a shotgun bride? Or because I looked like I was hiding a medicine ball under my mini? The Spanish word for pregnant is *embarazada*. I usually felt pregnant and proud, but this time embarrassed was closer to the truth.

At home I changed immediately and was surprised to see that I had holes in the heels of my panty hose. Was I that leaden? The ten pounds I was carrying was equal to a bag of kitty litter, no more, no less. And lately I avoided carrying anything else. "A woman in my condition," I'd say to Rob, savoring the words, "can't be expected to take out heavy garbage."

Fall was here and my pregnancy was keeping me toasty warm. Sometimes when Rob and I went walking, I'd surprise us both by offering him my scarf or oversize jacket. It was hard to believe that our baby was due at the tail end of autumn. That we'd soon be taking family walks. How well would we adjust?

In my teens, I'd baby-sat day and night and usually loved it — the toddlers and the money. In my twenties, kids didn't do a thing for me — except get in the way of adult conversation. Now that I was thirty and six months pregnant, I was trying to slowly open myself up again to the charms of children.

Rob and I spent a weekend with our neighbor Andy, his very

pregnant wife, Nancy, and their almost-three-year-old son. After dinner, Max crawled into Andy's lap. Instead of thinking, "Is that kid still up?" I felt a pang of tenderness. In the morning, we were awakened by male whispers: "What color sneakers do you want to wear?" "Blue. I love blue." "You know what I love? I love Max and I love Mom." Instead of thinking, "It's seven A.M.!" I thought "Awww."

Pregnancy was making me soft around the edges. Literally.

I haven't done any exercise since you guys made me stop jogging," I confessed to Dr. Romoff. "I haven't even played my Jane Fonda tape."

"That's okay. Your normal level of activity is high. And having a tape is like taking homework on vacation — you don't do it, but it shows good faith."

I also said that I was still sleeping on my back. A book I'd read said I should be sleeping on my left side and warned that sleeping on one's back could squash one's intestines, aggravate backaches and hemorrhoids, inhibit digestion, and interfere with breathing and circulation.

Dr. Romoff shook his head. "That stuff is important in a complicated pregnancy, but yours isn't complicated. A woman can sleep however she wants, and in the overwhelming majority of cases, things go fine."

"What about bending or stretching too much and tangling the umbilical cord?"

"Nature protects the fetus. It's okay to bend and stretch."

I thanked him, closed his door, and was setting up my next appointment when Liz, the nurse, came in with late-breaking news about my urine sample.

"You're spilling a little protein."

So much for going home cheerful and reassured. I didn't know what to ask. I didn't want to hear about blighted ova.

"Can it be corrected?"

"Yes."

"If it's really bad, what is it?"

"Preeclampsia. But it's probably dietary. Or a fluke. Come back in two days and we'll check it out again."

I took the crosstown bus and gnawed on a cuticle.

The password was preeclampsia.

I looked it up in Sheila Kitzinger's *The Complete Book of Pregnancy and Childbirth*. "If mild preeclampsia goes untreated, eventually protein appears in the urine. Babies of mothers with a high proportion of protein in their urine may be born prematurely; once a woman is excreting a lot of protein, her pregnancy is unlikely to continue for longer than two more weeks. . . . In its severest form, preeclampsia becomes eclampsia, and then it can seriously affect you as well as the baby, causing convulsions and possibly a state of coma."

Was that a coma I felt coming on? No, I didn't think so. I told myself not to be an idiot.

I called Dr. Romoff.

"We had such a pleasant talk," I said, "and then Liz found protein in my urine."

"It comes and goes in pregnancy. Don't worry about it."

"It's not preeclampsia?"

"It's not preeclampsia."

"Okay. Thanks."

I liked having an easygoing doctor. But what made him so sure anyway?

Two days later it was determined that the protein scare, like the hormone scare, had been a false alarm. One that, once again, made me cradle my stomach and feel relief, gratitude, and exasperation — at modern medicine and at myself.

I vant to take your blood," said the woman with thick accent, thick glasses and a pink kerchief on her head.

Because my father had had diabetic tendencies, I was told I needed to sign up for a special glucose tolerance test.

"My name is Zebab," the woman continued. "You like Coca-Cola?"

"No." A dermatologist forbade it in high school and I'd never reacquired the taste. My Uncle Tom, a Texas banker whose claim to fame was having been locked in his vault by Bonnie and Clyde, drank a bottle every morning until he died at ninety-one.

I looked away as she straightened my left arm and inserted the needle. "Now we talk," she said.

Shoot now, ask questions later.

"Have you fasted?"

"Yes."

"Drink this. It's not Coca-Cola. Maybe you like."

She handed me a ten-ounce bottle of Trutol 100, a caffeine-free carbonated soda. Disgusting. I wished they had donuts, a Danish.

She handed me a card marked 10:00, 10:30, 11:00, 12:00, 1:00. My, we had quite a morning ahead.

By noon I had downed two bottles of soda, given blood four times, and peed in four cups.

"Can I go out and buy a sandwich? I'll be back before one, and I swear I won't eat anything."

She consulted with her higher-ups. Did I look like the type who would run away? Who would pig out on a sundae and not tell?

Inside I felt the pitter-patter of restless feet. My baby was either starving or on a sugar buzz.

They let me leave. By 12:50, I was back, tuna sandwich in tow.

One more needle and I'd be outa there.

Rob was about to leave town for ten days to direct an industrial film. I was secretly looking forward to the calm, though I wondered how I'd survive even a short absence once we had a baby to take care of.

While he packed, I ran a few girls' names by him.

"Page?"

"Eh."

"Leigh with a *gh?*"

"Too contrived."

"Zoë?"

"She wouldn't be able to leave New York City."

"How about Victoria and we'll call her Tory?"

"Nah."

"How about something Russian like Lara or Natasha?"

"Nyet."

"How about Abracadabra Ackerman and we'll call her Abby?"

"Nope."

How about Zebab? I thought. "You know, if we ever have a girl in May," I said, "we can name her May. April if she's a preemie, June if she comes late."

Rob zipped up his bag.

So far, I liked the name Elizabeth and he liked Katherine. For a middle name, we could borrow Davis from my family or Warren from his. But I still hoped to come up with a name that was neither common nor complicated.

We were better prepared for a boy. We'd decided my last name would be his first name, and we'd call him Wes.

But Wes what?

Weston William Ackerman, after my dad? Weston Kenneth Ackerman, after his? I felt I deserved an extra vote since the baby was getting Rob's last name. He didn't see it that way.

Meanwhile we were learning once again that trying out names on family and friends was risky business. Most of our ideas were met with vehement vetoes, indifferent shrugs, polite nods, or the occasional "Why?" Maybe such comments were helpful, but if we ended up overriding a parent's or friend's objection, we'd offend them for sure.

Back to the books of alphabetized lists. Picking out names was not as easy as A-B-C.

What does an almost seven-month-pregnant lady do for entertainment when her husband is away? Gets out her little black book and calls up single males. I had dinner with Seth one night, with my writer friend Masello the next.

"I'll have a beer," he said to the waitress, then turned to me. "You want one? Oh, you can't, you're pregnant."

"Some women think one beer is okay," said the waitress.

"Yeah, but she already had three scotches before we got here."

I considered ordering a Virgin Mary but didn't want to invite any immaculate conception jokes. I asked for a grapefruit juice and a mushroom cheeseburger.

"I hear rare meat isn't good for pregnant women either," the waitress offered. "Shall I make it medium-well?"

"Sure." I'd have preferred medium but didn't want to be accused of child abuse.

"So, you working on anything interesting — besides waiting for contracts and contractions?"

"This is my real work-in-progress." I patted my belly. I was enjoying my professional hiatus, but I still felt defensive about it. "I'm giving a talk soon at a prep school about combining career and family," I added. "They picked me because I'm the only roly-poly teen writer they could think of."

Our drinks arrived. "Here's to a roly-poly baby," he said.

"Cheers. Last week someone called to see if I wanted to write a book called *The Parent's Guide to Child Safety.* I said no. I was afraid it would make me paranoid, and between moving and having a baby, I'll have my hands full."

I asked Masello if he liked the name Weston Warren Ackerman.

"Yes," he answered, lifting his beer. "But the kid will have to become President."

Would I want my child to be President? I wondered the next day at my neighborhood coffee shop. Would I want my son or daughter to have to work that hard, to be constantly in the limelight? Every mother must hope her child will meet with success. But I didn't want to lose mine to a cause, however noble. I didn't want him or her to become a slave to the single-minded pursuit of more, more, more.

What did I want? I wanted my child to grow up happy. And since life can be wayward, I wanted him or her to have enough good luck and good sense to keep happiness forever within reach. I hoped, too, that my child would always feel comfortable talking things over with me. Someday soon over apple juice and hot chocolate; someday later over wine and coffee.

That's what I wanted. I wanted my child to be my friend. I wanted to pass the torch to a friend.

A man sat down alone at the next table and interrupted my reverie. "Eat here often?" he asked and began talking about local restaurants. He was starting to flirt and I didn't know how to let him know that he was wasting his time without embarrassing him unduly. So I did the polite thing. I didn't get up until he'd said good-bye.

With Rob gone, I made a brief getaway of my own. Five college roommates had organized a reunion in Vermont. On the way north, I stopped at a gas station and asked for directions to I-95. "I hope you're not driving alone," the man said. "You shouldn't drive so far when you're pregnant."

I still didn't mind the overprotectiveness of waitresses and gas station attendants. In small ways, the whole world was looking out for the next generation. And no, I wouldn't be driving alone. Ellen would be going with me. But six hours in a car is a lot. When we arrived, I felt as though the baby had hunkered down inside me, staking out new terrain. I wanted to stand on my head and shake it back up.

"Look how big you are!" Amy said when she saw me.

"I know. I'm jumbo. I'll be even bigger tomorrow."

Whenever we all got together, at a wedding or reunion, it felt like an episode of *thirtysomething*. We'd been friends for a dozen years, and we each wanted to hang on to the bond of our interlaced pasts. We no longer shared the world of classes, dorms, and dining rooms. But we still wanted to orbit around each other, and we were willing, when necessary, to forge through an occasional awkward conversation if it meant the knot of our friendship would hold, that the braid of our bright college years would not unravel.

We cooked and ate, walked and talked, read and played Trivial Pursuit.

"Should I get my tubes tied?" Helen asked, looking up from the Sunday crossword puzzle.

There was a silence.

Helen was married to a man fifteen years older and seemed convinced that neither of them wanted kids. Sonia was married and had a son. I was married and pregnant. Ellen, after a long courtship, was about to be engaged. Sally and Amy were single.

Sonia finally spoke up. "Life and love are fragile," she said, "I'd wait." The rest of us nodded in agreement.

The next day, as Ellen and I were getting ready to drive back, someone called me to the living room. A bumpy blanket was spread across the coffee table, but I didn't put two and two together until everyone yelled "Surprise!"

Underneath the blanket were a huge white teddy bear, two Beatrix Potter books, a Maurice Sendak wild thing, a handmade wooden rattle, and a pair of socks with elephants on them.

I was touched, and again jolted from nostalgia into reality. In college, Helen had been much more maternal than I; she was always the favorite baby-sitter of faculty families. Yet it was I who was expecting: expecting a baby whose hands would hold these toys, whose feet would fill these socks.

When Rob came home I caught him up with the news. "Susan's period is overdue," I said, "and she's guardedly ecstatic." I was, too. For her and because it would be great to have a close friend with a baby. "And a Wall Street guy made a decent offer on our apartment, but then reneged before I got it in writing." I was the wheeler-dealer in our couple and was miffed about this fish that got away.

I'd quickly called back some of the realtors I'd begun to call off. One said her client, the pediatrician, would be overjoyed, that *he* had been "brokenhearted" that he had let our apartment slip through his fingers. This time he came through with an offer of his own, but it was $10,000 below what we wanted. I decided to stall.

The next day a wonderful thing happened. A musician and his wife showed up, fell in love with the place, and said they could match the Wall Street offer. Chanda nestled between them, purring and twitching.

"We have an old cat, too," said the musician. "I see yours doesn't groom herself anymore either." I didn't take offense. He was looking compassionately at Chanda's matted fur and curling claws, and he told me that they had to constantly brush their cat and clip his claws.

I liked the idea of this couple and cat picking up where we left off. "We have a deal," I said, and we shook on it. "I hope we'll be able to move quickly. I'm in my third trimester. I'm not getting any smaller."

Rob could hardly believe it when I called him at work.

Neither could my lawyer. "So it's not the Wall Street guy or the pediatrician?" he asked.

"No, it's a musician and his wife. Kenny and Amy."

"Well, don't sell it to anyone else tonight." He laughed. "Now spell their last name."

Oh, God. "I didn't get their last name. But I have the realtor's card."

"I hope you know what you're doing, Carol."

"They like cats," was my feeble reply.

A week later I got a call from the pediatrician's mother. She said her son was very upset to have lost our apartment twice. Was there any chance it was still available?

"I don't think so. We have signed contracts."

"You are going to be a mother," she said in her heavy German accent. "I am a mother. Children cease to be children, but a mother never ceases to be a mother."

I felt terrible. I wished I had another apartment to offer her kindhearted slow-moving son. And I was sure I'd screwed up my karma for good.

Water dreams.

I dreamed Robert masturbated in the bathtub and his sperm turned into glistening goldfish.

I dreamed I was playing in tidal waves and felt exhilarated but also scared.

I dreamed I had a son who lay facedown in a shallow pool and needed to be turned. "You got me into this," he said. "You get me out."

They say pregnant women have weird dreams. Maybe it's because we are gluttons for sleep. You sleep for two; you dream for two. "And you have a lot of water sloshing around inside you," Rob pointed out.

And inside that water? More and more people were placing their bets.

"A boy," said Inez, who cleaned our home every two weeks. "You're kind of pointy."

"A girl," said Karen, who worked at the ob/gyn's. "But I'm always wrong."

"You're going to have *un varoncito*," said the elevator man. "And I'm always right."

"You're going to have a gorgeous girl," said a painter I passed on Broadway and Eighty-third.

"Think so?" I smiled. Construction workers had been ignoring me lately. My wide girth had rendered me invisible. I used to tense up when I walked by a road crew because I was afraid they might say something. Now that I was seven months along, I'd hurry by because I was afraid they might not.

"Yes, ma'am," he said. "Six pounds seven ounces."

Sometimes Rob voiced a preference for a girl ("because little girls adore their daddies and we won't have to fight so much during adolescence"). But he also liked the idea of a son. A son who, he imagined, would look like him, root for the Yankees with him, tinker around the house with him.

I had a feeling I was having a boy. Why? Because I was carrying high versus low, out versus around. And, crazy though this sounds, because Rob and I both come from boy-first families. Having a boy first, to blaze the trail and protect the siblings, seemed to me the American Way. A shamefully sexist view, to be sure, but when I grew up, I liked having big brothers who could not only keep me out of trouble but introduce me to guys who could get me into it.

I called an airline to ask about flights to Boston over Thanksgiving and told the woman on the phone that I'd be in my ninth month. She said it was okay to fly until seven days before one's due date. Before signing off, she added, "I hope it's a little girl."

"You do? How come?"

"Because little girls are made of sugar and spice and everything nice, and little boys are made of snips and snails and puppy dog tails."

I was glad we weren't on some futuristic T.V. phone because I rolled my eyes. But a girl would be great. I was the girltalk maven, after all. Whenever I went window-shopping at baby stores, I was spellbound by the Mary Janes and smocked dresses. And lately, I'd begun to notice mothers walking and laughing with their grown daughters. I remembered the old adage: "A son's a son 'til he gets a wife; a daughter's a daughter all her life."

A friend of my mother's asked what I thought I was going to have. "I'm beginning to think a boy," I said and stopped just short of saying, "But it doesn't matter so long as it's normal." A near faux pas: her daughter has cerebral palsy.

I told Rob about this conversation. He confessed he'd become much more receptive to solicitations from March of Dimes, Special Olympics, Children's Research Hospital, Save the Children, Easter Seals. "Stuff I used to consider junk mail, I now read thoroughly. Last week I got a letter about cystic fibrosis and how some girl called it 'sixty-five roses.' I sent them fifteen bucks. Normally I wouldn't even have opened the envelope."

I'd become a pushover, too. I'd just sent ten dollars to the School for Special Children simply because they asked.

I liked to think that if we had a handicapped child, we wouldn't become too frustrated with his or her limitations. I liked to think that we'd become the kind of parents who'd say, "He's given me more than I've given him," or "She's taught me more than I've taught her."

Yet would we? Would we be patient enough? Selfless enough? We'd have no problem loving a handicapped child, but would we be able to cope? People do. We would. But it was something we tried not to think about.

My publisher sent me the cover of *Girltalk About Guys*. On the back it read that Carol Weston "lives in New York City with her husband and first child." The words worried me. I hoped we weren't tempting fate.

It was amazing to think that if the baby were born now, it would probably survive.

But, I thought, stay put, kiddo. Hang in there where it's nice and cozy. Get bigger and stronger and wait until we move. It'll be better, much better, for all of us.

At the post office, a man apologized for *not* holding the door open for me. At the bank, an ancient woman offered me her place in line. At home, I rested a book on my belly — and it moved. Sometimes it felt like a barroom brawl in there; other times it felt as though the baby's toes were stuck in my rib cage.

By now I no longer climbed stairs unless necessary. I hesitated before stooping for dropped coins, pen caps, even ice cubes. I no longer felt self-conscious wearing a dress with sneakers — although if the sneakers came untied, I needed help tying them back up. And according to Rob, I was given to much sighing and grunting.

My mother and Lewis returned from Cape Cod. She was taken aback by my profile, impressed by the round-the-clock belly dance beneath my shirt. The baby was fluttering and thumping, doing fetal calisthenics. And I'd never seen Mom looking so brown, girlish, and well-rested. Once hard-driven, Mom had had an idyllic summer. "I scarcely made any headway on my writing projects," she confided, "but it's hard to type when you're holding hands."

With just two months to go, I still held out hope that babysitting and hand-holding would mix a little better.

Time was, Rob and I would go to the movies, he'd put his hand in mine, and we'd whisper sweet nothings. Now we'd go to the movies, he'd put his hand on my belly and I'd whisper, "D'ja feel those flip-flops?"

We'd chosen a ten o'clock showing of a film the critics called, "sizzling, steamy, and scorchingly sexy."

I'd started yawning before it began. "I doubt I'll be feeling hot and bothered when we get back home," I'd told Rob.

And I didn't. But he did.

"It's twelve-thirty," I protested. "I don't want to."

"A quickie? It's been almost a week."

"I'm eight months pregnant as of yesterday. And I warned you. I don't have it in me right now."

He put my hand where he wanted it to be. I removed it.

"I said no. I'm exhausted."

"Will you tell me a story?" he asked.

Lord, help us, I thought. I closed my eyes and chose the path of least resistance.

"Once upon a time . . ." I began, then took a moment before continuing, "there was this beautiful young raven-haired waitress whom everybody lusted after. Her restaurant was always packed and men couldn't take their eyes off her gorgeous legs, ample bosom, and" — I really am a good wife, I thought — "taut little waist. One day, this fellow named Rob was having dinner there, and she leaned over and said, 'Hey, handsome, I'll be off in ten minutes. Any chance you can give me a lift home?' Well . . ."

In short, the gent accepts, she leads him to her bedroom, and on her black satin sheets, she proceeds to do unto him all the things I didn't have the energy for.

Moments later, the party was over.

"Thanks," Rob said, heading for the bathroom. He kissed me good night and laughed. "Phone sex with my wife."

I was asleep before he got back into bed.

We made a bid on an apartment around the corner. It was bigger than ours and was painted bright pink throughout. Even the ads admitted it needed TLC. But we'd fixed up places before, and if it meant getting a below-market price, we were willing to put in the labor.

Easy for me to say. My labor would come later. Rob would do the spackling, painting, and tiling, and we hoped to enlist friends for the actual carting of furniture. We couldn't see hiring a company, or even a truck, to take tables and chairs just half a block away. At the very least, we knew we could count on Ed. He and Beth lived in a five-floor walk-up and were eager to amass I.O.U.s before it was their turn to relocate.

My job was to oversee our sale, pay transfer fees, arrange for a safety inspection of the new apartment, secure a mortgage, photocopy W-2 forms, ask for letters of recommendation for the new co-op board, hire someone to sand the floors, and begin packing.

"And Rob, we can't keep putting off Lamaze classes."

I knew he wanted to wriggle out of this. Not fatherhood, but the miracle of childbirth. He hated that men no longer had options, that they couldn't get away with just pacing in the waiting room.

"I don't want to see you suffer," he said.

Oh, please. "I'm not looking forward to suffering either, but that doesn't mean you're getting off easy. I'll need you."

Thirty-five years earlier, when my mother had her first child, my father was neither invited nor missed in the delivery room. She didn't want him to witness the unseemly mess of childbirth. Mom took pride in looking pretty for Dad. She put on lipstick every morning, cologne every evening. She wouldn't have dreamed of borrowing his razor.

"Rob, you don't have to take along a catcher's mitt. You just have to be there. You can stay by my head, okay?"

I signed us up for Sunday-night Lamaze classes, the only ones I thought he'd be available to attend.

Alone I attended a midweek infant-care class at Lenox Hill Hospital that had begun the previous month.

"People are dropping like flies," one woman observed. "They must be already having their babies." She told Lorraine, the British instructor, that her doctor thought she was carrying a huge baby.

"Do you have big feet?" Lorraine asked.

"Size ten."

"Then you'll be fine."

I raised my hand. "There's a correlation between foot size and pelvis size? I have small feet — size five and a half."

Lorraine looked worried. "What about your wrists?"

I held them up. "Tiny — too small for bracelets."

"Well, just don't gain too much weight."

Gee, thanks. I hoped this was Old World folklore.

I settled back to learn about bathing the baby. "Warn your husbands that the umbilical cord is gross and awful, so it doesn't scare them," she advised. "Talcum powder may contain carcinogens, so use corn starch." "And don't be afraid of the soft spot on your little one's head." (Afraid? Who, us?)

We saw a Johnson & Johnson film featuring happy parents washing happy babies with Johnson & Johnson products.

In marched two new mothers to share their war stories.

Mom Number One went into back labor and said she was "begging for medication," then received so much that she "could have been anywhere on the planet." An overeager anesthesiologist misunderstood her doctor's orders and gave her a second epidural just when the doctor wanted her to start pushing. They had to yank out the baby with forceps "as big as salad servers" and yes, it hurt.

Mom Number Two was turned away at the hospital because she wasn't sufficiently dilated, so she and her husband took a

walk. On Park Avenue. Where she started groaning and panting. "My God, that woman is in labor," said a passerby. By the
time they got back to the hospital, it was too late for an epidural. The pain was "excruciating" but went fast. Then they did
an episiotomy, and some of the stitches opened up shortly
afterward.

Perhaps Oprah should sign these women on, I thought.

Lorraine asked if there was anything the women didn't have
at home that they wished they had.

"Diapers," said mom Number One.

"Hired help," said mom Number Two.

I told Rob about my afternoon, and he said he hoped the baby
would come early.

"Why?"

"Because I can't wait. And because then we won't have to
worry about when it's going to happen."

"Well, I can wait. Once we have it, we have it for life." Rob
was ready for a son or a daughter. I was content with just a
baby-to-be.

Was I a bad mother already? The baby was so much easier to
care for inside me than it would be outside. Pregnancy was a
piece of cake; I felt celebrated, special. And we could still go out
night after night. How would I feel when the baby arrived —
sweet but needy? When our social life ground to a halt? When
I got my period back and had to fool with birth control? I didn't
envy mothers who were loaded down with baby paraphernalia
and squalling children. I was still banking — banking — on
the rumor that when it's your kid, every sneeze is enchanting,
every eyelash a gift from God.

We had an early dinner with a college friend of Rob's who lives in Japan and whom he hadn't seen in years. Though not particularly pretty, she was a helluva lot slimmer than I was. Afterward, she planned to rush to the theater and we planned to cab to a party. I was ready to bid a fond farewell.

Maybe we should meet later and go dancing," Rob suggested.

"I'm not going to want to go dancing after the party," I said, and clawed his knee under the table.

"I will. Sounds like a great idea," she chimed. Bitch.

"You sure you won't want to come?" Rob asked.

"I'm eight months pregnant," I reminded him, bruising his shins with my heels.

"Okay, I'll pick you up at your hotel at eleven," he said, and we all pressed cheeks good-bye.

"You shit," I said as we taxied uptown. I hadn't forgotten that hers was the last pair of bosoms he'd squeezed as a single man. I wasn't worried about infidelity, but I didn't like the idea of their heading off to a club without me. And I didn't want to dance the night away with them.

At the party, a woman asked how far along I was. "Six months?"

"No, eight." I took it as a compliment. When I was four months pregnant and someone guessed six, I'd also felt flattered. Six must be the magic number: you're more pregnant than fat, but you're not yet a walrus.

Another woman asked if I was "due any day now."

"Any week," I corrected. She got flustered and said how terrific I looked one too many times.

Parents offered advice. "Talk a lot now because once you have the baby, you'll be talking *to* him or *about* him." "Put your dirty T-shirts in the baby's crib; he'll find the scent comforting."

"Buy white — not purple — grape juice until your kid is seven." "Change the baby's diaper in the middle of a feeding. If you do it before, he'll poop again; if you do it afterward, he'll be asleep."

Rob looked at his watch. "I gotta go," he said. "Sure you don't want to come?"

"And waddle my way through hordes of loud, drunken dancers? No thanks."

After he left I talked to my friend Masello. A woman congratulated us. "No, no. I take no responsibility for that," he said, pointing to my belly.

The hostess walked up. "Carol's water just broke," Masello whispered. "Can she use your bed?"

She went pale.

"Just kidding," he said, having shortened the woman's life a year or two.

An artist in his late forties eyed my belly and wished me well. I asked if he was a father. "I think so. I've lived in thirty-one countries."

I talked to Susan. She was thirteen weeks pregnant and tired of throwing up all the time. "And I'm a little worried because my last pregnancy ended around now."

"But last time, you weren't so nauseous, so undeniably pregnant, remember? For you, the morning sickness is a good sign, and it will subside pretty soon."

True enough, but I felt for her and for everyone for whom throwing up is a ruthless part of pregnancy.

"Susan, I'm about to turn into a pumpkin, and the baby's pummeling me from within. I'm going to take off."

I thanked the hostess and headed home alone.

Turned out I should have given Rob a curfew.

At midnight I was in bed reading and tossing out old magazines. Hey, no prob.

At 1:00 A.M. I was getting tired of flipping through *Mademoiselle*s, but I still felt fairly unruffled.

At 1:30 A.M. I was annoyed. I could handle his recent prepartum passion for rollerblading, volleyball, and boyish athletics, but this excursion was out of line.

At 2:00 A.M. I was ticked as hell.

At 2:15 A.M. I left a nasty note outside our door and turned off the lights. The note read, "I've lost all respect for you." Chanda and I settled into bed, and as she purred, I smouldered and wished I'd written, "At hospital having baby. Regards, C." I stayed mad and hoped the baby didn't pick this moment to develop its nervous system.

At 2:30 A.M. the phoned jarred me awake. "Hi! I didn't want you to worry. We're having pizza, and I didn't want you to think I was in an accident or anything."

If Rob imagined he could unload his guilt that easily, he was sorely mistaken. I hung up on him, tossed, turned, and finally found my way back to sleep.

At 3:30 A.M. in walked Prince Charming himself.

"I knew I was already in hot water," he mumbled, "so I figured I might as well make the most of my last night of irresponsibility."

"Screw you," was my reply. I didn't want to talk about it on one hour's sleep.

The next day, after hurtling rough words his way, I forgave him. He was appropriately contrite and I believed him when he said the evening had been platonic. Besides, we were sealing our marriage with a child. I didn't want to go to divorce court pregnant. And deep down, I understood his final fling with freedom. I, too, might have enjoyed such a night if only I could have found someone who had a thing for oversize women, someone who would rather dance stomach-to-stomach than cheek-to-cheek.

Rob offered me a back rub and I accepted. We set up a donut

of pillows, I climbed in, and he began to massage. Minutes later, he was ready for things to escalate. "Uh, uh, buddy. This one's all for me. It's your penance." I shifted my weight. "A little lower and to the left, please."

My mother phoned. Something about the National Wildflower Research Center, for which she is a trustee. "We're going to a gala dinner tonight and I may not be able to take you to lunch after all," she said. It still baffled me that she seemed busier now, retired, than she was when she was a magazine editor. Lewis joked that she was as overbooked as an airline.

"Okay, Mom, but if we don't go out soon, you won't recognize me."

We made a date for the next day.

An editor from a teen magazine invited me to lunch. I must have been sending out hunger signals. A restaurant meal *is* the easiest way to down those dark green and orange vegetables.

I wriggled into my silk maternity dress and took the subway to midtown. Advertisements in the train read, "Pregnant? We can help," but no one gave me a seat.

At the restaurant, I greeted the editor and we sat down. My napkin kept sliding off my lap. I no longer have a lap, I realized, I have a lump.

Over pasta, the editor said she hoped to be pregnant soon.

"My pregnancy has been easy," I said. "I bet you'll sail through yours, too."

"I won't. I'll get sick."

"Maybe not. They say the chance of having morning sickness is about fifty-fifty."

"I'll get sick," she repeated. "I had an abortion and I was sick during that pregnancy."

"Oh." I tried not to gag on my gnocchi. "At least you know you're fertile."

She pitched a few article ideas and I was torn about whether to take one on or save these remaining weeks for the move. My list for that afternoon was to buy glazing putty, semigloss, and wallpaper, and to call the plumber, lawyer, and co-op board president. Why have a last gasp of professionalism now?

Maybe because I was afraid if I didn't, I never would again. Part of me knew that life was long and that it was okay to be a postmodern neotraditionalist — to take time out to smell the diapers. But part of me also knew that my identity, for better and worse, was tied up in my career: I write, therefore I am. I agreed to write an article for teen girls, "Why I Act Like an Idiot in Front of Guys I Like." She agreed to give me a flexible deadline.

For the first time in seven years, Rob took my address book to work. For the first time since the Easter after my father's death, Mom invited me to church — three Sundays early. And when she and I finally had lunch, I mentioned my friend Valerie and Mom said, "Give me her number, will you? I really should have it."

Something was up.

"If someone is throwing me a shower," I said, "we should talk them out of it. I got gifts on my birthday. It's too much." I felt lucky enough to be great with child, why should my child-less friends have to fete me and spend money on me?

Mom turned colors and spilled the beans.

I tried to talk Meredith and my cousin Laurel out of it. I tried to talk Caroline and Seth's girlfriend Lucie out of it. But they insisted and said the presents wouldn't be for me, they'd be for my baby.

So I resigned myself to feeling grateful but guilty.

I was now going to the ob/gyn's every two weeks instead of every three.

Liz listened to the fetal heartbeat. "Strong baby."

Dr. Yale felt my belly. "Perfect."

I beamed. "Think my navel will pop out?" By now, it was neither inny nor outie, just sort of stretched flat.

"I doubt it," she said, "but I make no guarantees. How is everything else? How are you feeling?"

"Fine. Large. Slow. Tired. We're incapable of going to bed before midnight, so we feel like sleep-deprivation experiments already and the baby isn't even here yet."

Every night at eleven, I'd say, "Rob, let's go to bed," and he'd say, "Okay," but then we'd keep on puttering. Seems we both needed a parent to bark, "Lights out!" We were two grown kids staying up past our bedtime night after night.

"You need your sleep."

"I know. Fortunately my seventeen-year-old cat, who is usually worse than a newborn as far as yowling all night, sleeps better now that it's cold out." I'd been inadvertently getting revenge on Chanda. I was now disturbing *her* two or three times a night so she'd move aside and let me go to the bathroom.

I told Dr. Yale that I'd noticed a little milk — colostrum — on my right breast. "Just a drop." I'd noticed it not during a shower or sex, as my pregnancy books had foretold, but when I was going over the galleys of my manuscript.

"That's okay," she assured me.

Okay? I knew it was okay. I was looking for a gold star, a pat on the back, a small parade.

I took the bus back home, wondering if now that my body was hidden in a winter coat, I'd gone back to looking dumpy rather than pregnant. Apparently not. A woman offered me her seat and I was pleased to accept.

Her civility proved contagious. Another woman, about forty, offered an elderly man her seat. "Thank you for the seat, young lady. I appreciate it," he said. "Thank you for calling me young lady," she replied. "I appreciate it."

A few stops later, a mother and her baby sat down next to us. The baby clutched my index finger, gripping it for several blocks. "Adorable baby," I said to the mother.

Yes, I wanted one. But I still wanted to move first.

"When are you due?" she asked me.

"December seventeenth, and I hope it doesn't come any sooner."

I didn't know whether to cross my fingers or my legs.

Ninth month, homestretch.

We still hadn't moved. We were in the throes of picking out carpeting for my office, selecting window treatments for the apartment, removing brass hardware from doors so we could paint, and pleading with the co-op board to please accept our buyers so we could get the show on the road.

Was childbirth like moving? So difficult and overwhelming that you swear, "This is the last time," until, a few years later, you find yourself at it again?

Rob and I ordered Chinese take-out for dinner. His fortune read, "You long to see the great pyramids of Egypt."

"Bad timing," I said. My horoscope that morning had warned, "Watch those pounds!"

We flagged a cab to Lenox Hill Hospital for our first Lamaze class. I half expected the driver to race us across town, but he just drove at the usual reckless Manhattan speed.

We knew we had found the right room when we saw nine other Buddha-women and their partners. Our instructor, Deedee, a little woman with a big voice, asked how many of us had felt Braxton Hicks contractions, "a sneak preview of things to come." Nearly everybody. She explained cheerfully that the irregular tightening of the uterus will become more common and eventually go from "mild to painful to very painful to overwhelming to excruciating to unbearable. If you're among the unlucky 25 percent of mothers who have back labor," she continued, "it will hurt even more."

When she called a five-minute break, the women made a beeline for the ladies' room. The men — our "coaches" — were told to grab mats and pillows so they could help us learn how to relax and go limp.

I tried to remember why I'd been so adamant about signing us up.

Lamaze was supposed to teach couples how to stay in control of the biggest event of their lives. Lamaze was supposed to enable them to make informed decisions about drugs during childbirth. Lamaze was supposed to help husbands and wives bond before their twosome became a threesome. Lamaze was supposed to lead to enduring friendships with other new families.

Lamaze was not supposed to scare you silly.

The second class was also unnerving. Perhaps it wouldn't have been if we'd been meeting in someone's comfortable living room. But I'd signed us up for the cut-rate hospital course. The overhead lights were bright; the chairs were cold and stiff; the education was graphic.

Deedee described the preliminary signs of labor: dropping, increased vaginal discharge, and the "passing of the mucous plug, a pink, brown, slimy thing." Many women get a "spurt of energy," she said, "and go from laid back to keyed up, which means labor may be a day or two away."

One husband looked at his raccoon-eyed wife and said, "A spurt of energy? That will be a blessing." The rest of us laughed. Had this been *The Newlywed Game,* she'd have bonked him on the head with an oak tag card. But she looked too exhausted even to scowl.

"Then you have contractions," Deedee continued. "And true labor begins."

We women shifted in our seats.

"Don't call your doctor unless your water breaks, contractions are coming regularly for an hour, or you bleed — which would not be a good sign."

A drill sergeant in nurse's uniform, Deedee showed little mercy. She described labor as climbing hills, scaling Mount Everest, and dodging volcanoes. "Now my mothers will swear and say, 'Leave me alone,' but coaches, don't you dare. She'll say, 'I can't do it,' but you can help her do it. You can grab her shoulders and make eye contact and breathe with her. Afterward many of my mothers say, 'I never could have made it without Steve or Tom or Ray.' Now that would make me feel ten feet tall."

Nobody looked convinced.

Finally she did a crash course on breast-feeding. Breast-feeding, judging by the beatific expressions of the mothers (especially Mary) in Renaissance paintings, seemed easy, natural, and downright idyllic. Not so, according to Deedee. At first it's awkward, painful, and doesn't quite work. Kind of like sex for virgins, I thought, knowing what a rude awakening intercourse can be for my teenage pen pals.

"How many of you were breast-fed?" she asked. Only two women raised their hands. "And you all turned out fine. Remember that if you run into problems."

She offered helpful tips and showed us a short film depicting tens of mothers — and scores of breasts. The camera zoomed in on a tiny sleeping baby, born five weeks early. Its mother was saying how hard it would be to leave the hospital empty-handed. But I was thinking, five weeks? Five weeks? Is my baby already that cute, that whole?

Party time. Meredith and Laurel's featured pink and blue balloons, bouquets of baby's breath, and plastic infants stuck in cheeses and cakes.

One friend asked if we had a beeper in case I went into labor while Rob was on location on some shoot. God forbid. I hadn't even thought about that. Meredith said, "You could always leave a message on your answering machine saying, 'Rob, rush to the hospital!!! Everybody else, leave your name, number, and the time that you called.'"

Meredith suggested a party game and assembled a ball of string and a pair of scissors. "We're all going to try to guess how big Carol's waist is," she explained. I, by now a veritable exhibitionist, stepped into the middle of the room, lifted my shirt, and did a 360.

One by one, guests cut pieces of string while I opened presents. I usually feel self-conscious in front of a stack of gifts because I'm afraid I won't be able to ooh and aah over each with equal grace and sincerity. But every baby item — the lullaby mobile, the teddy-bear quilt, the bunny clock, the miniature long johns — was so adorable that the exclamations came on their own. One advantage of waiting so long before having a baby, a guest joked, is that your friends have more money and can give more generous gifts.

I didn't know about that, but I did feel a glow among my friends that day. Some were new friends; some were school friends; and some were second-generation friends — our mothers had been close in college. I hoped that mine would be the first of many baby showers celebrated together and that it would be followed by rounds of children's birthday parties, and perhaps, decades from now, by weddings, more showers, more children, more friendships.

And how well did everyone guess my waist size? Meredith wrapped a string around me, snipped, and handed over the master piece to measure against all the estimates. Ellen was just two inches off. Jen was off by an insulting eight inches. Patty had cut an extra foot. "You were supposed to guess my waist, not my height," I said. But by the time I'd gone around the room, I found that nearly everybody had overestimated my girth. Even my mother allowed for an extra four inches of belly. Meredith alone came in three inches under the mark.

"How come you came in under?" I asked, suspicious.

"I cheated," she confessed. "My sister taught me this game and said the trick to winning was to guess what you think, then lop off thirty percent."

Caroline and Lucie's party was also a grand success. It began as a tea and shower for the ladies. At seven o'clock, cups and saucers were replaced by wine glasses and hors d'oeuvres, and husbands and boyfriends began crowding the room.

One friend's mustachioed fiancé asked if we were nervous or excited about the big moment ahead.

"A little of both," I said.

"It should be fun," Rob said.

I glared at him. "Fun?"

"I bet labor will be a snap for you."

There was — forgive me — a pregnant pause. Which I broke. "You'd probably tell a draftee that war is an adventure," I said. "I don't think 'snap' is the word you're groping for."

My, but the guest of honor was touchy. The mustachioed man slunk off, and Ellen took his place.

"Last night I dreamed Rob got the flu, and I had to deliver the baby," Ellen said. "It was a girl."

"Really?" I told them a story I'd heard about a woman who, upon giving birth, asked her husband, 'What is it? What is it?' But all he could answer was, 'It's a baby! It's a baby!'"

Ellen spoke of her sister, the wild child. "My parents didn't have to raise her; they had to tame her." She turned to Rob. "I trust you have my name on your list."

"List?"

"List. The husband brings a list and a roll of quarters to the hospital so he can call everyone."

That list. We made a mental note to start collecting names and coins.

My pregnant friend Arlene and I talked about discovering bathrooms in stores that we'd been going to for years. Someone else asked if we'd thought about schools yet. A businessman acquaintance confessed he'd dreamed his wife had a baby and he'd faxed it away. A woman who grew up in Manhattan said we should tell our child that F.A.O. Schwartz is a toy *museum:* a white-lie tradition among city parents.

At eleven, when Rob and I returned home, we were zombies. I put pillows under my head and stomach, and prayed that Chanda would let me sleep through the night.

Deedee guided our Lamaze class through the hospital maternity ward. "If you come in before midnight, you'll be charged an extra day. So use your judgment, but hold out if you can. Remember how long labor usually takes."

She pointed to a door on the sixth floor marked Father's Waiting Room, then eyed the men. "You won't be out here, fathers. You'll be in there with my mothers."

She showed us the labor room, which featured an amni hook (for breaking the water if necessary) and a spiral electrode (a sort of thin corkscrew that could be inserted into the vagina and attached to the baby's head). We all recoiled. "It isn't pretty," she agreed, "but it monitors the baby's heartbeat in a clear beep beep beep. The external fetal monitor makes the heartbeat sound like a posse coming down the road."

Next she said that each woman in labor could have just one coach — husband, mother, sister, friend — not two. Just one? At first I felt disappointed for my mother. Then I realized she might feel relieved.

We filed by the delivery room ("where my coaches will wear scrubs, a shower cap, a face mask, and booties"), the recovery room, and a postpartum room.

"How about the ladies' room?" I asked. She pointed.

"Does the ward get extra busy during the full moon?" Rob asked.

"You better believe it," Deedee replied.

A woman whipped a calendar out of her purse and said, "That's December fifth this month." I vowed to spend that day in bed, reading, writing, resting, napping. Unlike many of the women in our group, I still wasn't ready for the grand finale, the big beginning.

Last stop: the nursery. We peered through the glass at rows of bundled babies. Some newborns were crying (I thought,

Nurse, do something!) but seemed composed moments later. Others were sleeping like angels. Rob squeezed my hand. Would our baby really be here in just a few weeks? It was both exhilarating and sobering to imagine.

Deedee also showed us the room of Isolettes for sick babies, but nobody chose to look or linger.

Tuesday I woke up charged. "Get out of bed," I snapped at Rob. "I want to wash the sheets. Besides, it's not fair for you to always sleep more than I do when I'm nine months pregnant."

Rob buried his face in the pillow. "I'm the coach," he mumbled defensively.

"Get out of the shower," I barked moments later. "I need to wash the towels."

He peered at me from behind the curtain. "Is this your spurt of energy?"

"Bite your tongue," I said.

But there was no slowing me down. After the laundry, I went Christmas shopping. I normally despise those efficient people who check everyone off their list before mid-December. Yet this year, I knew that if I didn't shop before I dropped, I wouldn't shop at all.

A saleswoman rang up a sweater for my father-in-law. "Good luck," she said. "Everything changes once the baby is born. But remember: your husband comes first — men are babies, too."

More and more people were offering unsolicited advice. I didn't object. I just didn't take it to heart.

At the ob/gyn's, I had my first internal exam in months. Dr. Yale inserted a lubricated gloved finger into my, a-hem, birth canal, and announced, "You're about 40 percent effaced." I was astounded. She said that was normal and that any dilation and effacement (thinning and shortening of the cervix) that could be accomplished painlessly would get me off to a head start for labor. She also wished me a happy Thanksgiving in Boston, and said to call if I had a "bloody show."

Gee, that sounded festive.

At the Andover Inn on Thanksgiving morning, Rob and I made love. Not with abandon. With care and caution and too many thoughts ricocheting between us. First I felt sentimental: my family, the three of us, was right here, safe together. And Rob felt extra loving: there was room in me for all of us. But then I grew uncomfortable and worried that the baby was already coming between us. And Rob got nervous and worried that we might induce labor.

Sex was making us think too much.

The Rolling Stones verse, "This could be the last time, maybe the last time, I don't know," played in my head. At some point Rob and I would have to go from a sex life that was cut back to one that was cut off.

"Honey, will you bring me a glass of water?" I asked. Even half asleep, Rob knew I was nearer to the sink than he was. But rolling out of bed was not what it used to be. "It'd be an opportunity to show your love," I added in pear-shaped tones.

"Didn't I just do that?" he asked groggily.

We drove to his sister Lisa's to celebrate with Rob's family, grandfather, in-laws, and new niece, Sarah. Rob marveled at her "sweet smell" and how well she sat up. He tossed her in the air and she giggled adoringly. She was seven months old, a good age. Responsive and beyond the blob stage, yet manageable and not into everything.

I could see that my niece was hands-down cute, but I wasn't aching to tickle her. I still wasn't receptive to the magic of babies. Was this unnatural? Or was my lack of zeal more typical than some pregnant women are willing to admit?

Gene, my mother-in-law, asked if I was ready to have a baby. "No."

"She wasn't ready to get pregnant either," Rob said, "and she took to pregnancy like a duck to water."

Quack, quack. Who knew? Maybe he was right. Maybe it was just the labor of love that I wasn't ready for.

"Just keep that suitcase packed," Lisa warned. "And do your breathing exercises. They really help you ride through labor — one contraction at a time. Remember, too, that the pain has a purpose."

A purpose, I repeated as I lowered myself into the sofa next to Rob. I could feel the baby swooping and diving, each kick another hello from the future. Rob lifted my shirt. "Dad, get a load of Carol's stomach!" he said, and my belly performed on command, bulging and rocking.

"That's amazing!" Rob's sister Sally said.

"I'm glad I was born too early for all this crap," Ken said and got up to get a drink. "I didn't have to be there when Gene hatched her babies either."

I smoothed down my shirt. The peep show was over.

"You want a Bloody Mary?" he asked Rob.

"Sure. I'm drinking for three."

Lucky Ken. He had a father, a son, a grandchild. Rob's immediate family was intact, untouched by tragedy. I knew that Ken had a soft side, and I hoped he appreciated how much family, good family, surrounded him that day. Four generations of his blood.

Sarah rolled over on the floor and giggled at her grandfather. "What's your name, kid?" he asked. "Can I pick you up by the ears?" He chucked her under the chin and she laughed.

When the holiday was over, I hugged him good-bye. "I guess we won't see you before we have the baby."

"You won't see me right afterward either." Ken prided himself on his ability to combine business with pleasure, and would undoubtedly finagle a meeting in New York as a pretext to come see his new grandbaby. Even on our wedding day seven years earlier, he conducted some first-thing-in-the-morning business.

Lisa loaned us "Womby Bear," a battery-operated teddy bear

that mimicked the sound of the womb. She said it had been a great source of comfort to her baby. We thanked her for it and for the weekend.

"Good luck!" she called from her front door. Gene was going with us to help get things ready for the move and for the baby. "Bye, Mom. Wave bye-bye, Sarah." Sarah curled her tiny fingers and opened them again.

I adjusted the seat belt around my bulbous belly. Part of me did kinda feel like a draftee going to war.

That Sunday night Rob and I attended our last Lamaze class. Gene came with us and took along her knitting — a green-and-yellow baby blanket. Several couples were missing, and no one knew if they were feasting and toasting or panting and pushing.

Deedee started right in. "Don't have false expectations," she said. "During labor, your coach will be with you constantly, your nurse will be there every fifteen minutes, and your doctor will check in every two hours."

She showed us the "pelvic rock," which was supposed to relieve the pain of back labor. It sounded more like a dance step.

"Drugs won't take away the pain, but they will take the edge off. The problem is they can make your baby sleepy and listless, and if the doctor says 'Push!' you don't want to say, 'Push what?'"

Drugs. I liked knowing they were there as a fallback, but Rob hoped I'd be able to have the baby without them. Rob, who had no qualms about getting high in college. Rob, who couldn't begin to go nine months without beer. Rob, who even now didn't hesitate to open a bottle of wine with dinner though he knew he'd be drinking alone.

Do men undergo vasectomies without drugs? No. Most men refuse to undergo vasectomies at all. Most let women get their tubes tied, even though that procedure is more complicated, more expensive, and less-easily reversed.

Drugs. I wished Rob didn't care so much. What was so noble about natural childbirth, anyway? This wasn't California.

Deedee told us to practice our breathing: the Sniffle ("as though you have a cold"), the Big Blow ("as though you're blowing out a candle"), the Quick Exhalations ("hee hee hee"), the Startled Breath ("huh!"), and the Cleansing Breath (what was that again? I was getting mixed up). She walked around the room listening as we, the swollen-bellied, inhaled and ex-haled in unison.

"Okay, we're going to do an experiment," she said. "Coaches, I want you to squeeze my mothers' arms as hard as you can — no cheating — and mothers, I want you to breathe." Our eyes went wide. Were Lamaze classes more touchy-feely in the seven-ties — or in the heartland? Where had we gone wrong? "Now!" she barked. I sniffled and hee-hee-heed as Rob squeezed as hard as he could.

"Who could have tolerated more pain?" she asked.

Most of us cautiously raised our hands.

"Good. Now coaches, try it again, and mothers, don't do your techniques."

Rob squeezed and it hurt like hell. A chorus of "Ouch!" "Stop!" "Quit it!" and "That's enough!" was heard around the room. "You squeezed that hard last time?" I asked. He nodded. "We better start practicing our breathing," I said and he agreed.

Next we got to hear about cesareans. "They're necessary when the baby's head is bigger than the mother's pelvis, when the fetus is in distress, when the mother has diabetes, active herpes, or toxemia, when the mother's waters have broken but she's not making any progress, when the baby is a breech birth . . ."

I let myself space out. The room was hot and I was zonked. I knew that of the nearly four million babies born in America each year, almost one in four is delivered by C-section. But my doctors weren't cesarean-happy. Their practice had a low rate of C-section deliveries and I hoped this part of the lecture wouldn't pertain to me.

". . . In seconds, the mother is put to sleep; in minutes, the baby is removed. The doctor uses a staple gun to sew her back up." Rob and I squirmed and I tuned out again, the way you stop looking when a movie gets too gruesome.

I wanted to believe that my labor, in the ironic words of my ob/gyn, would be uneventful. I prayed it wouldn't be a life-or-death situation. No, I didn't want to lose my baby, but that baby was still a stranger. If one of us had to die on the operating table, I didn't want it to be me either. I wondered how long after childbirth the selfish survival instinct defers to a mother's fierce love and willingness to sacrifice. Immediately? After one week? Two months? More? I looked at my mother-in-law. Gene would die for Robert.

I massaged my belly. It was getting tighter in there. But despite what my pregnancy books said about the baby getting settled and snug, I still felt a lot of poking around of hands and feet. I hoped my baby wasn't sitting on its placenta, using the umbilical cord as a necklace, or planning to emerge with its lungs clogged with meconium (a fancy word for baby poop).

At last, the moment Rob had been waiting for since the first class. He'd heard that expectant parents cry every time they see a child being born, and now we were finally going to get to watch The Movie, considered something of a classic.

"Childbirth is the hardest work you'll ever have to do," said the narrator as the music soared at full volume. On the screen, couples with long hair, bell-bottoms, and pointy-collared shirts talked about love and "the beautiful experience of childbirth." Then, as advertised, two mothers gave birth before our eyes, with, as Deedee put it, "their legs wide open so we could see the stage." Both times, right on cue, Rob and I started weeping.

"More blood than I expected," I whispered.

"Yeah, but not as gross." He said he couldn't wait to cut the umbilical cord — to launch our little ship. I kissed him. I was proud of his new attitude and I wished I were as eager as he. But I had a bigger part in labor, and my enthusiasm was tainted with anxiety.

"Before I hand out your graduation certificates," Deedee said, "Let me tell you what to take to the hospital." My pen was ready. "Socks, pillows, Chap Stick, a hand fan, tennis balls and a rolling pin in case of back labor, mints and lollipops for the mother, sandwiches for the coach, and a split of champagne for both when it's all over." Toasting to a healthy baby, now that was a moment I was looking forward to.

With that, she wished us well. Many of us exchanged phone numbers, but I doubted we'd ever really get together.

"So what did you think, Mom?" Rob asked as we caught a cab outside the hospital.

"I learned more than I ever wanted to know," she said.

Me too. And I wondered if I'd even remember those breathing techniques when the pain heated up.

Rob phoned from Ben's Babyland, a store whose motto is "We deliver when you deliver."

"Do you care what color baby bumper we get?"

"What's a baby bumper?"

He said it was a cushiony thing that goes around the crib. Gene had already shipped us the crib Ken had used when he was a baby in Lima, Ohio. Not only did it have character, but it discredited once and for all Ken's sister's assertion that my father-in-law was born middle-aged.

"I trust you and Gene to make a good choice."

"Are rabbits okay?"

"Rabbits are fine."

When they came home, they showed me a California Kids Sunny Bunny Blue Bumper, a white diaper pail, a yellow KangaRockaRoo, and a wooden rocking chair.

"We still have to get a stroller," Rob said.

Not to mention diapers, bottles, pacifiers, and a million other indispensables.

At noon, my mother joined us and we tried to work up some apartment-moving momentum. But with both moms around, Rob and I regressed pathetically. He moaned that he shouldn't have turned down a day of work for this and became suddenly paralyzed and overwhelmed. I sniveled that it wasn't fair for him to get overwhelmed when I had even more reason to get overwhelmed and we couldn't both be overwhelmed.

We were a study in how not to move. Clothes still hung in closets. Drawers were still full. Many of our packed boxes were marked "Miscellaneous" or "Surprise!" and contained everything from magazines to coffee mugs to costume jewelry.

I threw out shoes with worn heels and socks without mates. I stuffed pants and shirts into bags, but thought, was I ever this small? I began setting more and more aside for Goodwill.

Ed and other friends arrived. They rolled our furniture onto dollies, took it down one service elevator, wheeled it across the street, and took it up another service elevator. I knew it was generous of them to help us move, but it felt as though they were hauling off pieces of our nest, our life. When they came to tackle my office, I wanted to cry, not thank them. I felt like barring their way, throwing myself in front of my computer or file cabinet. I hated to transfer junk — yellow news clips, old correspondence, scribbled notes for unwritten novels — from one home to another. But it was too late now to sift through item by item.

Meanwhile, the phone kept ringing — faraway friends clamoring for news. My California friend said I sounded out of breath. "Getting up is hard work," I explained.

"So the baby's still hanging in?"

"Poor thing's probably learning stress management in utero. If it knows what's good for it, it'll stay put at least another week." I said that except for the tension of the move and the holidays, it'd been a good nine months and I'd had an enjoyable pregnancy.

"I remember having my head in the toilet bowl most of the time," she said, "but I loved it, too."

One friend called and said she dreamed I had a boy. Another said she dreamed I had a girl. I'd dreamed I gave birth, but my ob/gyn was falling falling falling, and I barely managed to cup the baby's head and break its fall. I'd also dreamed I gave birth to a baby *and* a cat, but the baby died, and I blamed the nurses for not reminding me to breast-feed.

Speaking of cats, Chanda was as strung out as the rest of us. She didn't approve of all the commotion and meowed nonstop, demanding to know where people were taking her sofa, her bed, her pillows.

I had decided, somewhat guiltily, to have her spend a few nights alone in our nearly empty apartment while we fixed up the new one. She wouldn't have liked the mayhem, and besides, I needed at least one good night's sleep before Labor Day. I put out lots of food and water and positioned blankets in all the prime sun blocks. Then I apologized and promised to visit several times a day.

That evening, as Rob and Gene moved tables and chairs around the new apartment, I worked on the baby's room. The Baby's Room. I emptied shopping bags of shower gifts and lined our shelf with teddy bears and Peter Rabbit books. I hung up yellow-striped stretchies, a mint green gown, and a pair of red thermal long johns.

The hangers were little. The outfits were little. There was a full yard of empty closet space between the clothes and the floor. It was all so unbearably cute it took me aback. I called Rob and Gene to take a peek, and the three of us marveled at how clean and sweet everything looked, including the empty crib that stood ready and waiting. The afternoon's frustrations gave way to a warm tide of maternal feelings, and rather than fight it, I welcomed it.

Gene flew back to Columbus, and Rob and I spent our first night alone in our new home.

In the morning Meredith came by to lend a hand. Boxes upon boxes were everywhere. "So have you consummated the place yet?"

"Does this look like a boudoir?" I asked. "Rob wanted to, but my consummating days may be over."

Then again, maybe not.

Ten . . . nine . . . eight . . . seven. My due date was one week away and I had an ob/gyn appointment at eleven o'clock. I poured myself some cereal, got out the milk, and was startled to notice that the expiration date on the carton came *after* my baby's projected birthday.

"Week thirty-nine," Liz said as I stepped on the scale. I hadn't gained any more weight, though I certainly wasn't holding back on Christmas cookies.

She listened to the baby's heartbeat and checked my abdomen. She frowned and checked again, pressing this way and that. "This mound up here? It's the head. You have a breech baby, my dear."

A sonogram confirmed the unsettling news.

"We've been moving and I guess the baby has been moving, too." I tried to smile, but the tears were already on their way. "Don't mind me," I sniffed. "I've been a crybaby all week. I'm just exhausted. I know it's not the end of the world." Liz handed me a tissue and put her hand on my arm. "What's the percentage of breech babies?"

"Three to four percent."

Dr. Yale came in and prodded my belly. "My husband was a breech birth," I told her.

"It's not genetic and it's not because you've been lifting boxes. The baby was just trying to get more comfortable."

I hoped it had succeeded. That would make one of us. "It *has* been active all week. It's been like a Rockettes audition in there. I just can't believe it decided to do a somersault now." Little athlete. Little moron.

She mentioned the possibility of version, in which doctors gently nudge the baby around. But sometimes version sets off labor. And the success rate was better before the very last week. They decided to check the baby's mobility.

It had just done a back flip. How stuck could it be?

Dr. Romoff poked my belly. It hurt and the baby didn't budge.

Pretty stuck, apparently.

"If my nerves weren't so shot," I said, and pitched another soggy tissue into the wastebasket, "I wouldn't be crying so much."

"Well, it is upsetting," Dr. Romoff replied.

Wait a sec. He was supposed to be Mr. Reassurance. "But only because I don't get to try for natural childbirth, right?"

"Right. Just because I'm commiserating with you doesn't mean you should worry more!" He explained that C-sections can be easier on the baby but involve more hospital and recovery time for the mother. He also said that in the past, breeches were often delivered vaginally, but sometimes the head got caught, and pulling the baby out could cause damage to the spine, nerves, or skull. "Every old-timer has one disaster story to go with his success stories, and in cases like these, I'd rather section a hundred women and deliver a hundred healthy babies, than deliver the same number of babies vaginally and wind up with one who is seriously injured."

Dr. Romoff said there was no reason I couldn't give birth vaginally next time.

I nodded and reminded myself that the important thing was to have a baby, not an experience. But please, please, no more surprises.

"So does this mean I'll deliver on my due date?"

Yes. In one week, the baby would be, as Shakespeare put it, from my "womb untimely ripped." In one week, we'd be parents.

One week. Seven days. How many hours was that?

"What if I go into labor before Thursday?"

They didn't think I would. I wasn't any more dilated or effaced, and the baby's head was no longer putting pressure on the cervix. And if I did? I had their phone number.

My last office appointment was scheduled for Tuesday evening; my C-section for Thursday morning at 8:45 A.M. "May I use the phone?" I asked.

I called Rob. He said he loved me and pointed out that at least it wouldn't be a frantic cesarean after endless hours of labor. Better an "elective" C-section than an emergency one. "And the baby won't be a conehead. So what if it doesn't know up from down?"

Still, we were both disappointed. Months ago, Rob had felt squeamish about participating in our baby's birth, and I'd been terrified about labor. But, Lamaze had left us, if not eager, at least willing to give natural childbirth a try. Now it felt as though we'd completed the course and done all our studying only to be told there'd be no final exam.

I called my mother. She listened sympathetically and said it was probably a good sign that the baby was already standing on its own two feet.

No more hoping the baby would come late. I had to get cracking. I answered teen mail and finished my article for the teen magazine. (Amazing how fast I could work when I had no time to procrastinate.) At home I looked up cesarean in my pregnancy books and read that the mother should cough and move after surgery and that recovery can take six weeks. I wondered what else Deedee had told us while I'd been daydreaming. I retrieved Chanda. It was her last week as our only baby and I wanted her by my side and purring.

When Rob came home, he kissed me, greeted Chanda, and waved his index finger in front of my belly. "Now listen, kid," he scolded. "You're too old for this kind of carrying on." Poor chickabidee, a disappointment to his parents already. Rob speculated that maybe it had scrambled around after hearing about the spiral electrode, that baby corkscrew.

"At least I won't have to have an episiotomy." I told him that the Lenox Hill policy — since changed — was not to let dads into the operating room. Frankly, neither of us minded.

Gene called. "Do you want to come Friday?" we asked. No, she did not. She wanted to come Wednesday.

So be it. Why should Rob pace alone? We invited both grandmothers-to-be to the hospital so everybody could pace in formation.

The phone kept ringing and I told callers about the baby's shenanigans. Lisa blamed it on Rob — "Like father, like baby" — then, at the end of a pep talk, added, "I forgot to tell you to buy disposable nursing pads. When you hear a baby cry, your boobs leak. And when you're nursing on one breast, the other gushes along trying to keep up. Be sure to pick some up."

Seven days. Seven days.

Major surgery I could probably handle. Motherhood still had me panicked.

On Friday we closed on "Chanda's Place." It was high time.

That weekend we unpacked by day and saw friends by night. "When are you due?" men and women asked as they raised fluted champagne glasses at Christmas parties.

"Thursday at eight forty-five," I'd reply, then try to gauge just how uncomfortable I'd made them. The men invariably darted to the bar for a quick refill. The women offered their own or their friends' childbirth stories, both happy and frightful. Seems some women collect pregnancy and labor horror stories the way others collect recipes.

Rob came with me for the final checkup, presurgery consultation, and sonogram. Dr. Romoff showed us the four chambers of the baby's heart (a pulsing glob) and the two sides of its brain (a circle with a line down the middle).

No, it hadn't flipped. Yes, we were still on for Thursday at 8:45.

Dr. Romoff said not to eat or drink anything after midnight Wednesday and to go to the hospital two hours early. There, nurses and attendants would shave me, draw blood, and give me an I.V. Rob could be with me until I was wheeled away for the epidural and actual operation: a "bikini-cut" C-section. (The vertical variety got phased out around 1960.)

"You'll be hurting Thursday and Friday, but Saturday may be a turning point. You'll probably want just parents that first night, not a whole slew of relatives." He sat up in his chair. "No sex for six weeks."

"Can we have sex tonight if we want to?" I asked.

Rob raised his eyebrows and looked at me. Dr. Romoff raised his eyebrows and looked at Rob. "Sure," he said. No one dared smile.

"And it makes sense to have the operation on my due date, right? Tomorrow is Jane Austen's, Noël Coward's, and Beethoven's birthday. Maybe we should have gone for December sixteenth."

"When we know the due date, we usually try to stick with it. It depends too on the availability of hospital rooms." He stood up. "It'll all go fine."

We shook hands and thanked him.

"One more thing," he said. "Don't worry if I don't walk in until eight forty-six."

On Tuesday night Rob and I made love as best we could. It was hard to believe that because we loved each other and chose each other — because we had done *this* nine months earlier — we were bringing a brand-new person into the world.

"It's kind of daunting, isn't it?" I said, referring to my stomach.

"I feel like I'm doing push-ups." Rob laughed.

"There's more of me to love."

"There's more of you to work around."

In the morning I mumbled, "I dreamed we had a boy."

"I dreamed we had a girl," was Rob's sleepy reply.

On Wednesday we hung paintings, alphabetized record albums, touched up paint, paid bills, bought diapers and nursing pads, packed my hospital bag, and got our hair cut.

I wish I could say I was counting the hours until my baby's birth. But while I was excited, I wasn't in a mad rush to be slit and stapled.

On the other hand, I'd seen the pink up-and-down scar from Gene's cesarean. It began way up at her navel, and since Rob had been an upside-down baby, she had had to have cesareans for his younger sisters, too. C-sections may be too routine, but they're simpler than they used to be, and I knew I should look at the bright side.

Gene arrived, all jittery, and my mother called and invited us to dinner. Mom, too, was a bundle of nerves and sounded as if she'd been crying. "You okay?" I asked. No. Seems she thought I — her baby — would have to be knocked out completely. She was relieved to hear that a local anesthetic would do the job.

At the restaurant, I announced that we had finally sold the old apartment: "I closed on Friday."

"That's wonderful," Lewis said. "And you open tomorrow."

Rob and I laughed.

"How come you two aren't nervous?" Mom asked.

"Because you and Gene are taking care of that," Rob answered.

Thursday morning. We were wide awake when the alarm went off. We showered and dressed and I put on my watch. It read 6:45. According to the clock, it was only 6:20.

"What time is it?" I asked, and Rob checked his watch.

"Six forty-five."

"I can't believe it! We're late!" Rob had fixed the bedroom outlets the day before and had apparently forgotten to reset the clock. "Hurry up! Get your shoes on!"

I coated my nails with clear nail polish and blew to make them dry faster. "You doing your breathing?!" Rob asked.

"No, I'm doing my nails!" I said, and suddenly wondered why. In a minute one of us would probably start boiling water. "Let's go!"

I pressed the elevator button and Rob went running back inside for his coat. He couldn't find his key, so I locked up. When we reached the first floor, Rob realized he'd forgotten his list of people to call. I stepped out and handed him my key, and he headed back to the eleventh floor.

I flagged a cab. "Lenox Hill Hospital," I said, "but I'm waiting for my husband."

"Is he sick?" asked the driver.

"No. I'm having a baby."

His eyes appeared in the rearview mirror. "You seem pretty calm."

"I am," I said. "But wait till you see my husband."

Part Two

Birth Days

At the hospital, I was ushered into a wheelchair and taken to the sixth floor. Nurse Imelda checked my temperature and blood pressure. I liked her Caribbean accent and gentle manner. If I had to get shaved and give blood, I was glad she'd be the one wielding blade and needle.

She hooked up the fetal monitor and the room suddenly warmed with the sound of our baby's heartbeat. Gullumpgullumpgullumpgullump. As Deedee had promised, it was a posse of charging horses, richer than music. Rob and I listened and smiled at each other.

Imelda put me on an I.V. "When will the anesthesiologist do the epidural?" I asked.

"Soon," she said with slow island enunciation. "He's a very fine doctor. A real crackpot."

"Crackerjack?" I mumbled hopefully.

Rob took out his video camera. "How do you feel?" he asked for posterity.

"Psyched. Nervous. Cold." I was wearing only a hospital gown and green knee socks and I wished the liquid trickling through the I.V. could have been mixed with hot tea.

"Hear that?" Rob said as he panned the room with the video camera. "That's your heartbeat, little baby."

"Think the grandmoms are here?" I asked.

"I'd bet the co-op on it."

He walked to the waiting room, where, he told me, Gene and my mother both leapt up, ready for news.

But there was no news. And when Rob returned, Dr. Romoff came in and announced, "We've been bumped."

Bumped? As in airplanes?

A woman in labor needed an emergency C-section and Dr. Romoff had a laparoscopy to do at ten. My 8:45 surgery was rescheduled for 11:45.

I felt colder, hungrier. We'd been going full speed ahead for weeks and didn't know what to do with three anticlimactic hours. Take a nap? Call friends who might worry if they didn't hear from us by noon? Rob pointed his video camera at the clock. "You were supposed to be here by now," he said, dejected.

I rolled my I.V. along the floor and we joined our mothers in the waiting room. They leapt up again, but we told them to make themselves comfortable. We tried making small talk before the big event.

At 11:45, a nurse summoned us back.

"Drink this," she said. "It's oral citrate. Designed to neutralize stomach acids." I lifted the cup to my lips. "It tastes disgusting," she warned.

I threw it back. She handed me another.

Then she told Rob to kiss me good-bye.

It was time to get the show on the road.

I knew a C-section was the easy way out for my baby — and my husband. But what about me?

C-section. How quick I'd been to adopt that technical term, to cushion reality with the available padding. I told myself I was lucky to miss the experience of labor, lucky I wouldn't be flailing around like a fish on a hook.

Inside the delivery room, Dr. Verdier had me bend over so he could give me a shot in the back.

I didn't mind the bright lights.

I didn't mind being nearly naked.

I didn't even mind Rob's absence.

I minded the cold.

I was cold.

"Can't I wear more than this?" I asked as I lost all feeling in my lower body. "Aren't there any blankets?"

They had me lie down and strapped me to a table. A cloth barrier went up on my chest, shielding me from the goings-on below. "I'm cold," I kept saying, but no one came running with woolly scarves and sweaters. I asked a nurse to please hold my hands. And my feet? They were tingly, then numb, and I wanted to move them. It bothered me that I couldn't tell if I was wiggling my toes or not.

In walked Dr. Romoff wearing gloves and surgical attire. He was preparing to knead my insides, yet we exchanged pleasantries. Then he said, "You'll feel pressure but no pain."

I closed my eyes. Groan and bear it, I thought. He cut along my abdomen and I felt pressure but no pain. The dotted line seemed higher than I'd imagined, but I couldn't tell what was what.

Labor can take hours and hours. C-section babies arrive in minutes. A radio was turned down, but I could hear Stevie Wonder softly singing, "I just called to say I love you. I just called to say how much I care."

This was it. The big event. I could hardly believe it.

"You have a girl," Dr. Romoff said as he pulled out our newborn. "She's normal. She's perfect. She's beautiful."

I opened my eyes and saw my baby girl, my pink, wet, big-eyed baby girl. I'd been certain I was having a boy, but I was the only mother in there. This perfect girl was mine! A nurse held her up and I memorized her wrinkled face, her shiny body. I was so happy, so relieved. I was crying; she was, too.

"We have a girl," I told Rob over the hospital intercom. He was wearing a sterile suit, pacing outside the entrance of the delivery room. When the nurses handed the baby to him, he started crying. When he told Gene and Mom, they started crying.

Next thing I knew, I was in the recovery room, shivering and out of it. I asked Rob for kisses and details. "Six pounds four-teen ounces," he told me. "Born on twelve seventeen at twelve-nineteen, but I bet their clock is two minutes fast." A frank breech, he said, which meant that inside me, her fanny was down, her feet and head up. It also meant that now when she lay on her back, her feet rocketed skyward, an adorable idiosyncrasy that wouldn't last long, or affect development.

My I.V. bag contained pitocin to help my uterus contract. It hurt. The nurse came in and handed me our baby, supporting it as it tasted my breasts. Nine months of pregnancy hadn't quite prepared me for this first naked closeness, for these newborn kisses, for this remarkable baby that would become the focus of our lives and would someday call us Mom and Dad.

"What do we name her?" Rob asked. We'd both been so sure little Wes was on the way that we'd never officially agreed on a girl's name. Rob still liked Katherine and Emily.

"Elizabeth," I said, whispering my mother's stately middle name.

"Elizabeth," he repeated. He knew better than to argue with a woman with yellow-green skin and tubes in her arm.

At 3:00, I was rolled out of the recovery room and past the waiting room. The grandmothers, who had been there since dawn, popped out like cheerleaders to congratulate me and say they loved me.

And I, the new mother, the ailing heroine, smiled feebly, fluttered my fingers, and faded away.

I woke up in a postpartum room. I knew I'd had a girl, a normal, perfect, beautiful girl. But I was more focused on my terrible pain than on our wonderful news.

When we'd asked Dr. Romoff weeks earlier about the possibility of rooming in with our baby, he'd said he thought it was an overrated option, pretty in theory. Now I saw his point. I didn't want to have to deal with my baby. *I* felt like a baby: helpless, dependent, groggy, immobile.

A nurse came in and asked me to turn over so she could give me a Demerol injection to ease the pain. But turning over itself was painful. I gripped the bed bars and could scarcely move enough to expose one buttock.

I was thirsty and conned another nurse into giving me ice chips. Befriend the nurses, I told myself. Read their I.D. tags. Use their names. They're the ones who can provide relief every three hours.

While Rob and the grandmothers phoned family and friends, I dozed and moaned and waited for the next fix. No one had warned me that it would be like this. I wanted to feel waves of motherly love. But I wasn't even thinking about Elizabeth. I was thinking about Demerol.

I slept well Thursday night despite the nurses who wanted to take my pulse, temperature, and blood pressure. At first I resented their intrusions. But they also brought drugs. And they cleaned up. I knew about minipads and maxipads but had never experienced the monsterpads they used at Lenox Hill.

On Friday, Day Two, Dr. Romoff arrived and kissed my cheek. He'd been part of the biggest moment of my life and I was glad to add this new familiarity to our professional relationship. We had just been through the wonder of birth together and I wouldn't have wanted to revert back to patient and physician conducting business as usual.

I'd never forgiven my father's doctor for his clinical reaction when I'd called to tell him of Dad's death. He'd cleared his throat and defensively stammered, "That's the outcome we were trying to prevent." Jerk. I wasn't going to sue. All I'd expected was sympathy and human kindness.

Dr. Romoff removed my I.V. and told me I was about to have a breakfast of champions: tea, Jell-O, and apple juice.

"I'd prefer scrambled eggs, home fries, and a blueberry muffin."

He smiled. "Soon."

"And when will I have the strength to cradle my baby?" I asked and my voice cracked.

"Soon, Carol, soon." He put his hand on my shoulder. I still didn't trust myself alone with Elizabeth. She was frail and I was, too.

A nurse came to remove my catheter. I hadn't liked the idea of the tube being inserted, but I couldn't bear the thought of going to the bathroom on my own.

"Could I hang on to it just a little longer?"

She looked surprised. Was I the first ever to cling to the catheter? If so, how did others do it? I still could hardly turn over, let alone get out of bed and walk.

One of our pediatricians arrived. Rob and I had interviewed pediatricians together, as magazines said we should, and had chosen a team of three men — Levi, Kahn, and Traister — whose practice was a half block from our home.

"Elizabeth was a breech, right?" Dr. Levi asked. "She's got her legs in the air." He said I needed to nurse her every three hours for several minutes and to work up to about twenty minutes per breast.

With what energy? I wondered.

Rob walked in and said that even asleep Elizabeth was the cutest kid in the nursery. Little Miss Flying Feet.

I smiled wanly. I was exhausted and it was only 10:00 A.M.

The nurse came back and removed the catheter. With Rob's help, I hobbled, hunchbacked, to the bathroom.

Lunch was Jell-O and chicken broth. Gene, Mom, and Lewis came by during the twelve to one o'clock visiting hour. Gene brought photos of Rob as a baby. Everyone said Elizabeth was the spitting image of him. He beamed. I pouted. "Unfair," I joked, "after all *I've* been through."

Pain in childbirth. What had God been thinking of?

Gene also brought a white teddy bear wearing pale blue slippers, each featuring a rabbit's face and ears. It was for Elizabeth — but I cuddled it in bed that afternoon.

Lewis brought irises and said, "You've snapped back like a rubber band."

"I wish."

After they left, I thought about scribbling thank-yous, addressing birth-announcement envelopes, or reading the novels I'd carefully selected and packed. But there was no way. I got under the covers and collapsed.

I wanted — had expected — to feel unadulterated happiness. Our baby was here: healthy and whole. I knew how lucky we were that so far, our path to parenthood had been smooth, that I hadn't had to spend anxious months taking fertility drugs or anxious days in the intensive care unit for babies. And I didn't feel sorry for myself for having had a C-section. But I did feel guilty for feeling self-absorbed, for being as concerned with my body as I was about my baby.

Jen phoned. She could tell from my voice that I was feeling down. "What's wrong?" she asked.

"Why aren't I ebullient?"

"Because you just had major surgery," she explained.

I told her that I felt like a negligent mother already.

"Will you stop? You have your whole life to take care of Elizabeth. Right now you have to take care of yourself."

Mend first. Bond later. I thanked her and tried to nap.

Dinner was as hearty as lunch and breakfast. During the seven to eight o'clock visiting hour, Seth brought an azalea plant. It was good to see him. Rob and I had discouraged Thursday and Friday visitors, but despite my fatigue, I wanted, needed, to see friends.

At eight a nurse poked her head in and said visiting hour was over. Rob walked Seth outside.

"I hear you're doing great," the nurse said.

"Someone must be lying," I replied.

She asked to see my stitches and I showed her the five-inch smile from which Elizabeth had emerged.

"It's beautiful!"

"I bet you say that to all the C-sections." I blushed, and, to show off, shuffled down the hall to look in on my baby.

My baby. Mustn't forget I had a baby.

I also had a new roommate, a woman who had just had a C-section and was wailing and whimpering for Demerol.

Rob helped with the 10:00 P.M. feeding and Elizabeth found colostrum in both my breasts. I loved the feel of her suckling, but she was too heavy. I handed her to Rob, pointed to the bottle of sugar water, and had him finish the feeding, burping, and diapering. He was a doting dad: singing to her, petting her, wrapping and unwrapping her. He even filed her tiny nails because she'd been scratching her face. I videotaped them together.

"You know how they say, 'I wasn't born yesterday?'" I asked Rob. "Isn't it amazing to think that she was?"

We studied her, stared at her, hugged her, and tried to understand that we were parents now. That we had created this expressive little newborn, this miniature human being. Our baby. Our daughter. Our Elizabeth.

When we finally wheeled her back to the nursery, Rob put his sister Lisa's Womby Bear in the crib. I kept Gene's teddy bear for myself.

"Do you want us to wake you for the two and six o'clock feedings?" a nurse asked.

I shook my head no.

"You sure?" Rob asked.

"Sure." I couldn't rise to the cause. Not yet. I needed to regain my strength. Jen was right. Here, nurses would take care of her. At home, I'd *have* to do the night shift.

Not that I slept well anyway. My new roommate needed drugs as desperately and frequently as I had the previous night.

I offered words of encouragement and helped her summon the nurses.

And I realized I really was making progress.

Saturday, Day Three. Dr. Kahn, Pediatrician Number Two, arrived and escorted me slowly to the nursery. For a moment I wasn't sure if I'd be able to pick out Elizabeth — don't all babies look alike? I looked at the rows of newborns, like little papooses, and pointed to a small one with a Mohawk. Then I saw that its crib indeed bore Rob's last name. Dr. Kahn examined her and said she had a good heart, good lungs, good color. "And her legs are starting to come down." The morning feeding went well. I loved watching my daughter nuzzle hungrily against me, and I was glad she was doing her part to "activate" my breasts. The nurses even called her "greedy" before wheeling her back.

My ob/gyns walked in together. "You look fabulous," Dr. Yale said. "You don't look like you've been through surgery."

"I feel like I have." I chalked up the "fabulous" to their magnanimousness and to my having finally taken a shower. A nurse offered Percocet, but after spending two days hooked on Demerol, I was trying to wean myself from drugs. I didn't want to pass them on to Elizabeth, and I didn't want to be out of it when visitors came.

I wanted to be as exuberant as the mothers in the hallway, the ones who complained that it hurt to sit but who could walk briskly and breast-feed without pain. The ones who had good color and wore robes from home and, in some cases, even lipstick at visiting hour. I was still gray in my hospital garb and looked like I had applied one of those ghoulish white lip glosses that were popular when I was a teenager.

Friends called. "Good going!" said Norm, my next-door neighbor from childhood. "Max was breech, so Laura also got carved up like a Thanksgiving turkey. But she delivered Alex vaginally and it was a piece of pie."

Turkey. Pie. God, I was hungry.

Lunch was tea, Jell-O, chicken broth, orange juice. People always complain about hospital food, but I wasn't even getting hospital food. When a nurse saw the juice, she said, "You shouldn't have this yet," and took it away.

The indignity! I didn't mind being helped on with my panties or having to yank them down again whenever anyone in uniform asked to see my incision. But this was too much. I fought back tears.

"Take some Percocet," another nurse said. She was my favorite, the one most willing to move my phone closer, retrieve a fallen pencil, or offer other nonmedical help. And she seemed insistent. "Your milk hasn't even come in. Your comfort comes first."

I sighed. I hurt. I had gas pains. Enough of this bravery nonsense. Enough of this stoic waving away of modern medicine. Bring back the drugs.

"All right." I swallowed two pills.

Susan and Miguel visited that evening and took Rob out for a celebration dinner. When he returned to help with the 10:00 P.M. feeding, I said, "Just don't tell me what you guys ate, okay?" Would I have traded my firstborn for a doggie bag? No way. But I did ask an intern to ask my ob/gyns to please get me off this starvation diet.

Rob combed Elizabeth's hair with a pink baby comb that came in her crib along with a diaper and bottle of water. "She looks bigger than she did two hours ago."

"Think so?" We examined her delicate ears, her smooth elbows, the silken down at the nape of her neck, and the way her hair swirled at the crown. "And look at her tiny heinie!" I said and we laughed.

"Who does she look like? Me?"

"With a little of me thrown in." And a little of my dad, I thought, though I wasn't sure.

Rob and I took turns hugging and kissing our daughter,

drinking her in, beginning to connect. The nurse startled us when she came to say it was time for fathers to leave. Like a chambermaid intruding on a pair of honeymooners, she'd walked in on an intimate moment.

Sunday, Day Four. Breakfast included Cream of Wheat. I felt grateful beyond words.

I stumbled to the nursery to peek in on Elizabeth. Only one other baby was left in its crib; the others were with their attentive mothers. Elizabeth was asleep, smiling and fretting in her dreams. I blew her a kiss. Did I love her? Yes. More each day. Her floppy head that needed support. Her squinty eyes and innocent gaze. Her luscious cheeks and lusty stretches.

But it was easier to love her through the nursery window than to love her weight on my wound.

I ached, even with Percocet percolating in my blood. If I was this tired when I saw her only a few times a day, how would I manage at home? And what about bonding? Is it a one-shot deal? You get it right or you don't? If so, was I blowing it?

Dr. Traister, Pediatrician Number Three, came to my room. He told me Elizabeth had scored a 9 out of 10 on the Apgar scale, which tests a newborn's heart rate, breathing, skin color, muscle tone, and reflex response. Most babies score high, but I nonetheless felt a surge of pride — and gratitude. He also said to nurse her more often even if it were for less time. "Alternate which breast you start with."

"How will I remember?" Would it be like alternate-side-of-the-street parking, but without the helpful signs?

"Some women write it down and others switch a ring from hand to hand or move a safety pin around on their bra. Just keep nursing her or she'll get lazy," he warned. "Bottles are easier for babies." He also said I should nurse her in the middle of the night, if only for a few minutes.

I nodded and tears came to my eyes. From fatigue? Or from shame because I'd been shirking my duties? Letting the survival instinct beat out the maternal one?

Dr. Traister said we had to watch for jaundice, which is very

129

common in newborns. "Keep up the breast-feeding and give her lots of water. But don't worry. I'm not really concerned."

Well, I was. Jaundice sounded frightening. And when a nurse pointed out that Elizabeth was looking more yellow and that I needed to give her more water, I followed orders with a vengeance.

In fact, that's when I finally stopped focusing on myself and started turning my attention to my darling fragile daughter. I sat up in bed, held her close, and pushed her to drink whatever she could find in my breasts. I offered bottled sugar water, nudged her when her eyes began to close, and urged her to swallow more, more, more. "C'mon, lamb chop," I whispered. "I'll rally if you will."

First there was a drop of milk — real milk — on my left breast. I raced Elizabeth to it. Then there was a drop on my right breast. Quick! Elizabeth! Over here! Then, when she slept, I actually leaked. I couldn't wait for her to wake up and check this out.

But when she awakened, she wasn't interested. She just cried and cried and cried. A nurse came to wheel her away before visiting hour and I cried, too. Never had my breasts been so rebuffed, caused such disappointment. Even my Sunday supper — pot roast and potatoes — couldn't lift my spirits.

Visitors arrived for me and my roommate, but I couldn't wait until the next feeding. I was raring to go.

Yet by the 10:00 P.M. feeding, it was too late. My breasts were no longer just full, they were rock hard. Engorged. Useless.

A nurse suggested a hot shower before nursing. Another suggested hot compresses. A third suggested massage. Rob arrived, took one look at my silicone specials, and had ideas of his own. "Don't even say it," I said, wagging my finger. He retrieved Elizabeth from the nursery and she suckled valiantly. To no avail. The milk was stuck inside and she seemed unable to get at it. She and I both wept in frustration and I wondered if I *should* have enlisted Rob's help. I told him I'd try to nurse again at 2:00 A.M. and 6:00 A.M.

God knew why. The 2:00 A.M. feeding was a disaster. Nurses wheeled her in at 1:30, and Elizabeth and I made each other miserable until 4:00. Although I tried compresses and massages, and she smacked her lips and did all she could, I stayed engorged. A team of nurses offered advice but nothing worked. Finally Elizabeth was whisked away to the comfort of formula, and I was left behind with an electric breast pump.

I hated the loud aseptic machine that stretched my nipple like an udder. It hurt yet managed to extract only two ounces of milk. I handed over the precious vial and went to bed spent. I felt like a failed cow.

At 5:50 a nurse nudged me awake. I was sleepy and weepy and Elizabeth pulled and tugged for nought. I told the nurse to give her the milk I'd pumped. Defeated, I went back to bed.

Was I ready for the seesaw of motherhood? Were the joys and worries merely balanced? Or would I soon feel more elated than exhausted? I hugged the teddy with the rabbit-ear slippers.

Poor newborn baby. Poor post-op mom.

Monday, Day Five. The first pediatrician returned and said there was no sign of jaundice and that Elizabeth's weight loss (what weight loss?) was normal. He said to make an appointment to see him in one week. I told him about our hellacious night. "Your first days at home won't be a picnic either," he replied.

At 10:00 A.M., Elizabeth was more sleepy than hungry. She looked adorable, with her feet in the air and her big yawns, and I wanted to wake her so she could wake my breasts. I tried unwrapping her, tickling her toes, shaking her gently, changing her diaper. But even the nurses couldn't wake her. They wheeled her away at 11:30.

At least she'd be good and hungry for the 2:00 feeding. Sleeping Beauty. I wondered whether she'd still be sleeping in my womb if I hadn't had a due-date C-section.

The line, "Lady Madonna, baby at your breast, how do you manage to feed the rest?" ran through my head. Never mind the rest, how did she manage to feed the one she was nursing? And what about *getting* some rest? How did she manage that?

I heard from my Aunt Norah, my former roommate Helen, my friend Hannah. Hannah said her first baby weighed ten pounds thirteen ounces and was delivered vaginally. She must have told me that several years ago, but I was too ignorant then to be impressed. Now I was impressed.

Dr. Romoff took out my staples and replaced them with tape, so I no longer looked like I had a zipped-up abdomen. "Tomorrow morning," he said, "you're going home."

Ready or not, I thought.

At 2:00 P.M. a nurse rolled my baby back into my room. I'd already taken a hot shower and donned my new nursing nightgown, a pale blue number with two Frederick's of Hollywood slits stitched subtly down the front. I lifted Elizabeth and, yes!, she suckled. I was thrilled. She seemed pretty pleased herself.

As she nursed, I admired her red toes, long lashes, curls of hair, and jagged fingernails. I told her we were both new at this and that I'd be patient if she'd be patient.

At long last we were on track. Or so I hoped.

The next morning Dr. Yale came in and said not to have sex, drive, swim, exercise, use tampons, or lift heavy objects for six weeks. She also said it was normal that I was feeling dependent on pain pills. She gave me a prescription for Tylenol with codeine and assured me it wouldn't harm Elizabeth. (I looked up codeine in my Dr. Spock paperback and he concurred.) She also said to go back on my prenatal/lactation vitamins for two months.

One of our pediatricians came in and said we could go home. "When do I present Elizabeth to society?" I asked. I thought he'd want to ground us for two weeks minimum.

"Anytime. Just bundle her up and make sure the people you're with don't have a cold. If they're going to pick her up, make them wash their hands. And pay attention in the discharge class."

Discharge class? You'd think with all the oozing women wearing nursing pads and sanitary napkins, they'd have come up with a better name for the send-off course.

But Rob and I did pay attention. We learned how to swab the umbilical-cord stub with alcohol. And that a baby goes through six to twelve diapers a day. And that there was no need to set midnight alarm clocks — our baby would wake us.

The teacher also reminded us that women shouldn't take the Pill while nursing and that nursing is not a method of birth control. "Your periods may not return for six to eight weeks — more if you're breast-feeding. If applicable, you should be refitted for a diaphragm when the time comes."

Her parting advice: don't hover over the crib twenty-four hours a day; don't try to be superparents; and enjoy your babies!

Rob and I looked at each other. Were we really ready to venture forth on our own? Parenthood comes with owners' manuals — Spock, Leach, Brazelton, Kitzinger — but babies don't go by the book. Was I really ready to leave the hospital, with its call buttons, night and day nurses, and beds that moved up and down?

I weighed myself and was surprised I hadn't lost more of the weight I'd put on. Worse, my body was still misshapen: hard breasts, puffy belly, shaved mons. Oh well, who was looking?

We bundled our baby, gathered our things, and accepted the hospital's promotional gifts of formula, glucose water, lanolin, and A&D ointment.

A hospital volunteer carried Elizabeth, swaddled like an egg roll, to the front door. Rob hailed a cab and I told the driver to please drive very very carefully. As we crossed Central Park, Rob clambered into the front seat to get a better angle with which to capture our homecoming on video. I smiled wide, showed off Elizabeth, waved her little hand at the camera, and babbled something about the bun in the oven becoming a bundle of joy.

The cab pulled in front of our building and Rob held the flowers, bag, and camcorder, and opened the door for me and Elizabeth. I stepped out feeling like the President emerging from Air Force One. Passersby congratulated us. So did the doorman. So did the cab driver, whom we tipped profusely.

We were bringing our baby home.

It felt like a Norman Rockwell painting.

Part Three

And Baby Makes Three

Rob and I placed Elizabeth, fast asleep, in her crib and stood back to watch her breathe. She looked incredibly small and sweet, and I felt a rush of tenderness. "We did it," Rob said. "We made a baby." He offered his palm and I gave him five. We both leaned in and kissed her. Seemed we'd been kissing her nonstop since her homecoming. We were smothering her with affection now — before she grew old enough to protest.

Though we'd been home only a few days, gifts and cards were already pouring in. A stuffed elephant came with a note saying, "It's a jungle out there." A set of baby board books arrived with a Post-it saying, "These should come in handy — if only for teething." The mailman brought a bib marked "Spit happens."

One card defined *baby* as "a handy way of disposing of unwanted cash and filling up free time while cutting down on unnecessary sleep, curtailing a demanding social life, and curing a neurotic obsession with personal hygiene." Another said, "A new baby? Let us pause for a moment of silence — it may be the last one you get for a while." Still another card asked, "Why is a baby like instant coffee?" Answer: "It's easy to make and it keeps you up all night."

Elizabeth wasn't keeping us up *all* night, but she was making us rise and shine every few hours. She'd also resolved the question of whether we needed to buy a Fisher-Price nursery monitor. We didn't. Her room was next to ours and her cries came through loud and clear.

At first, Rob and I were dead set against pacifiers, those unsightly plastic plugs parents stuff in kids' mouths for hours on end. By our daughter's third day at home, we had a change of mind. Sucking after breast-feeding helped Elizabeth — and us — sleep, and we quickly realized that the pacifier was our friend. "Besides," I told Rob, "my mom patted herself on the back for never having given me a pacifier, but I sucked my thumb for nine years and bit my nails for twenty-three."

Because it was Christmastime, Rob's free-lance work was slow and he had lots of guilt-free time off. I still had trouble getting in and out of bed, and Rob was terrific about bringing Elizabeth to me, giving her sugar water, changing her, and cooking meals. I took photos of him bathing her atop a giant yellow sponge that filled our bathroom sink, and he took home movies of me singing her nursery rhymes and lullabies. On the stereo, he blared Handel's *Messiah*: "For unto us a child is born . . ."

Rob and Mom had also managed to unpack most of our boxes when I was in the hospital, so our home no longer looked like a warehouse. It was elegant and inviting and the lights on our Christmas tree sparkled merrily. I felt very fortunate.

I felt tired, too. I knew that with one efficient letter I could wish friends a happy holiday, inform them of our new address, send out birth announcements (our card read "Elizabeth War-ren Ackerman, 6 lbs 14 oz, and cute as pie"), and in some cases even thank them for a gift. But writing the letters was a hurdle I couldn't yet jump.

Days were spent taking care of Elizabeth and each other, and talking with well-wishers at home and on the phone.

And nights? What was nighttime now anyway? Short naps between nursing sessions. I was the milkmaid, the dairy queen. I was always on tap. I already felt if I could just have one full night's sleep, I'd be good as new. But when would that be? Weeks from now? Months? Years?

We'd been told we should rest when our baby rested, but that was our only time to get organized, to amass provisions. We tried to find easy ways out. We learned which stores deliv-ered diapers and groceries and which take-out restaurants offered the fastest, most nutritious meals. (City living has its advantages.) When friends said, "What can we bring?" we lost all coyness and answered, "A quart of milk" or "A corned beef on rye."

Mom and Lewis came by one night with the ingredients for pot-au-feu. We provided the pot and the *feu*; Lewis rolled up his sleeves and boiled chicken, sausage, turnips, brussels sprouts, shallots, and carrots. Dinner was delicious and the leftovers kept us going and grateful for days.

On Christmas morning we fixed them a champagne breakfast. Elizabeth wore a "Santa's Little Helper" bib and slept soundly through the festivities, trusting us entirely to keep her safe and warm, clean and fed. Her faith was not misplaced.

"Isn't she adorable?" I'd ask each time she settled into a slightly different position. "Look at her," I'd say when she nursed, her soft cheek on my breast, her noisy needy mouth finding milk where there had been none. I was unabashed, more maternal than modest. Breast-feeding was too natural, too lovely to hide from my family — her family.

Mom said she dreamed that Elizabeth was two months old and already talking. "You're so precocious!" Mom said she'd told Elizabeth. "What's precocious?" Elizabeth had answered.

"Precocious?" Rob interjected. "Nah. She's just like her Dad. She hangs out in a T-shirt, drinks heavily, and can burp on cue."

"How about you, Carol?" Lewis asked. "Are you feeling udderly tied down?"

"Udderly." I laughed, and moved Elizabeth from one side to the other.

Mom said she remembered as a girl asking her mother why men called women baby. "It's so demeaning."

"No, it's not," my grandmother had replied. "Babies are precious and soft and cuddly. Baby is a love word."

Rob and I didn't open our presents until Christmas evening. Normally we'd have ripped through all the wrapping paper by noon. But this year, the brightly boxed wine goblets, scarves, and colognes really did seem superfluous.

Elizabeth was our Christmas present. And tired though we were, having her at home was like falling in love all over again.

We weren't in the habit of eavesdropping, but the argument carried right through the front door. The couple across the hall had recently gotten divorced, and the ex-wife showed up in the hallway, unannounced.

"Talk to my lawyer. I get them on holidays."

"They're my kids too."

"Well you can't see them now so you might as well leave."

"I don't get support. You shouldn't get to see them at all."

"Will you keep your voice down?"

"Why should I? I don't have a pot to piss in. You cheap bastard!"

The son, five, cried, "Mommy! Daddy! Stop it!"

His little brother said, "Mommy! Don't go! I'll come out."

Rob and I looked at each other, horrified, fascinated.

"Let's never get divorced," he said.

"Deal," I replied solemnly.

Later in bed he told me I was looking sexy.

"Thanks. I'm not feeling sexy."

I was, however, pleased that my belly was subsiding, that my navel once again turned inward, that I was no longer hobbling as though I had osteoporosis. But I was still puffy around my incision. I still had to sport waist-high underwear and sanitary napkins. And I still didn't fit into my pre-pregnancy pants — even the ones that hung loose and that I was sure I'd slide right back into.

Worse, my nipples were sore. Now that Elizabeth and I had this breast-feeding thing down, she clamped on and suckled so furiously that I didn't see how I'd be able to keep it up every two or three hours. One of my nipples actually bled a little after a feeding. They also leaked when I heard another baby cry. And again when Chanda emitted a plaintive babylike meow.

"Doesn't nursing feel kind of good?" Rob asked as he snapped yet another photo of his wife and child at chowtime.

"I like it. I do."

"I read that some women get incredibly turned on by it."

"Where? In *Penthouse* or *Playboy?*"

"*Hustler*. In high school. It stuck with me."

"It's sensuous, I guess, but it's not erotic." I set a glass of milk down on a nursing-pad coaster. "Right now it hurts."

I knew it would get easier. But while our individual nursing sessions were often idyllic, there was — I hated to admit it — a certain relentlessness to the round-the-clock cycle of hunger and feeding. If I was tired at 2 A.M., I'd sometimes start worrying about how I'd manage at five. And eight. And eleven. There was no getting ahead.

"Imagine," I said to Rob, "if a woman performed oral sex on you every two or three hours with no break, no let up, for days and days and days. After a while you might want a breather."

"I doubt it," Rob said.

It was a bad analogy.

Elizabeth has lost more than the average amount of weight," said the pediatrician. "At six pounds five ounces, she's down nine ounces."

My eyes filled with tears.

"Don't be alarmed. But feed her more often, stop giving her sugar water, and bring her back in three days."

He explained that babies get 90 percent of each breast's milk in the first seven to eight minutes, so there was no need to wear myself out with longer feedings. "It takes the breast an hour and a half to fill up again," he added.

Why, oh why had we been plying our skinny baby with sugar water? They say you make all your mistakes on the first-born — that the first kid is like the first pancake.

Rob and I began a mission to fatten up our little titmouse. I nursed her in bed. In the rocking chair. In front of the T.V. I nursed while reading novels, talking on the phone, visiting friends. Rob helped bathe her, change her, and put her to sleep; I nursed and nursed and nursed.

One evening she woke up while we were having dinner, so I breast-fed Elizabeth while Rob fork-fed me. Sometimes she woke within an hour and a half, scarcely giving me a chance to refuel. Other times she napped for hours, and though we used to think, "Let sleeping babies lie," we now awakened her for her two eight-minute sessions, with occasional bonus minutes thrown in.

"Her cheeks look chubbier," Rob said.

"Our efforts are paying off," I agreed.

She did seem to enjoy the extra feedings. She'd either dive-bomb right on me or bump her open mouth against my chest, hit or miss, over and over, until she landed on her target. Then, having latched on, she suckled like there was no tomorrow.

One night at about three-thirty Rob nudged me.

"Elizabeth," he said.

"Huh?"

"Elizabeth," he repeated.

"Huh?"

"Elizabeth. She's crying."

"I have her right here," I mumbled, and pulled a small warm body close to mine.

"That's the cat," he said, and got up to rescue our baby.

The cat was worrying us, too. Chanda was gentle with Elizabeth and didn't seem overly jealous, but she was spending more and more time in her litter box. She'd had bladder infections before, but this was the first time she actually dripped on the carpet and sofa and bed.

"I'm scared," I told Rob and burst into tears. Much as we were enjoying these cozy days at home, much as we were proud of ourselves for managing without a full-time nurse or grandmother around, my nerves were thin, my tears at the ready.

I made a towel pillow for Chanda to lie on. Rob was worried about her, too, but he was just as worried about the carpet and sofa and bed. "We can't have two incontinent little animals in one household," he pointed out.

I decided not to ask him to take her to the vet. Though I still wasn't 100 percent, I also wasn't 100 percent sure he'd bring her back. So I bundled my nearly eighteen-year-old cat and walked to the Westside Clinic, petting her all the way, and wishing I could guarantee that our outing would be round-trip.

At the clinic an elderly woman was holding a thirteen-year-old Siamese who, she said, came in for chemotherapy every two weeks.

"You must be very devoted to your cat," I said, honking into a tissue.

"It's not my cat," she replied. "It's Roberta Flack's cat."

The vet called us in. He checked Chanda out, gave her a

shot, prescribed some pills, told me to phone in three days, and reminded me that Chanda was old — "not middle-aged."

I knew she was old. I knew I'd have to say good-bye to her soon. But I was glad I could put it off a little longer.

She may have been old. But she still purred when I petted her.

Chanda recovered beautifully. Elizabeth kept losing weight. We placed her naked body on the pediatrician's scale. "Five pounds fifteen ounces," he said. "She's down again."

We couldn't believe it. We'd been feeding her mercilessly — ten times a day. I looked at her and instead of seeing her long lashes and perfect nose, I saw how bony she was, how birdlike. The incredible shrinking baby.

"Give her more supplementary bottles of formula," the pediatrician said. "And Carol, have you been eating enough? A lactating mother uses up about the same calories as a construction worker."

So that was it. I knew nursing took it out of you, but I hadn't realized I'd been offering my baby skim when she needed cream. He put me on a diet of peanut butter, red meat, and whole milk. "Come back in two days," he said. "And on your way home, stop at the Häagen-Dazs on Eighty-fourth."

"You're kidding."

"No. Get a double scoop."

I stared at him.

"Doctor's orders."

Who was I to argue? At this rate, with exercise still out, I'd look pregnant again in no time.

Rob and I revised our mission: we now had to fatten Elizabeth *and* me up. At home he prepared a hearty meal of steak with pasta in cream sauce. We washed it down with milk shakes.

New Year's Eve and we were invited to a black-tie affair at our friend Caroline's parents' penthouse on Park Avenue. Elizabeth, now two weeks old, had already been to Cousin Charlie and Jeannette's for a cozy Christmas Eve (she'd slept in a carrier crib by their tree) and to Meredith's for a quiet supper (she'd slept on a blanket on top of Meredith's bed). But I considered this fancy evening her debut, her coming-out party.

I wriggled into a sleeveless gold lamé top I'd bought on sale and a black-and-gold hand-me-down skirt that I usually had to cinch with a safety pin. Rob donned his trusty dinner jacket and bow tie — he's the only guy I know who owns a tuxedo but doesn't own a suit. And since Caroline had sworn that Elizabeth was welcome, we dressed her in her most la-dee-dah stretchie.

"This is no pot-luck barbecue," Rob told Elizabeth as he pulled on her booties. "You'll have to be on your best behavior." I pressed a velcro bow onto a strand of her black hair.

At the party, she slept on Caroline's parents' bed in her carrier crib. She was oblivious to the toasts, singing, and friends who ducked in for viewings. Everyone said she was beautiful, and I beamed in agreement. At the buffet, I filled my plate three times but was so focused on Elizabeth that I could barely remember to ask friends about their jobs and vacations.

At one o'clock, our baby woke up wailing. We should have left sooner, but alas, we hadn't. I closed the master-bedroom door, scrambled out of my gold lamé, and got down to it.

Rob came in twenty minutes later to help change her. I removed her soaked diaper and he got a clean one. Too late! Elizabeth wet again — all over the Park Avenue bedspread. To laugh? To cry? I sponged madly with diapers and Kleenexes and Rob flung open drawers and medicine cabinets in a vain search for a hair dryer. Desperate, he started flapping the bedspread while I guarded the door.

Remarkably, the spot began to dry.

Once it had truly disappeared, we bundled up Elizabeth — now asleep and the picture of innocence — and began saying our good-byes. At the door, Caroline's mother clucked over our daughter — her serene face, her lovely baby smell — and regaled us with stories of bringing up her own three children. Then she thanked us again for bringing our baby along and having her be part of the celebration.

We returned to the pediatrician. Elizabeth had turned the corner: she'd put on five ounces. At six pounds four, she was still ten ounces shy of her birth weight, but at least she was heading in the right direction.

Me? I was getting more run-down. Maybe we *were* doing too much. Maybe we *were* seeing too many friends. But entertaining and going out kept our spirits up, and we didn't want to be just Mom and Dad — our other relationships mattered, too. Besides, friends not only got me through long afternoons, they also helped entertain Elizabeth.

I still couldn't seem to curb my expectations. It bothered me that I hadn't completed anything since Elizabeth's birth. I'd nursed and changed her, but there was more of that ahead. I'd sent out some announcements, but had dozens to go. I'd caught up on reading back newspapers, but new ones kept arriving. I'd eked out a few thank-yous, but more packages appeared. "Stop the presses!" I wanted to say. "Send back the boxes!"

Nothing I did stayed done and it was making me testy. When Rob voiced the slightest criticism, I'd cry. When, after a feeding, he said, "Elizabeth is still hungry," I took it personally, and brooded as he gave her formula. When he said, "Pretty soon you're going to have to help with the dishes and laundry," I sulked, though I knew he was right.

He was tired, too. And he hated when Elizabeth cried — even for a minute. He'd sometimes command, "Do something!" though he knew I didn't always have the answer.

I did, however, have the breasts, and he said he envied me that. But I envied him, too. Elizabeth and I could give him a night off. They couldn't yet do the same for me. Someday he might be able to slip her some formula, but now I'd get so full that I needed her at 4:00 A.M. almost as much as she needed me.

I did take a morning off, though. After a nine o'clock feeding, I stayed under the covers until noon and let Rob take Elizabeth to the pediatrician's to be weighed.

When they returned, I felt blissfully well rested. And they had good news: she'd gained a few more ounces. I kissed her ears and gazed at her rosebud mouth and the soles of her feet. I dressed her in her pink-and-white-striped stretchie and wrapped her in her pink-and-white-striped blanket. I picked her up, walked to the mirror, and admired our reflection. Mother and baby.

I rocked her in my arms and marveled that for nine months I'd rocked her inside me. Having a baby is a miracle, I thought, again and again for parent after parent. People tell you how tired you'll be, but they don't tell you that you'll also be drunk with love, on a high that doesn't quit. They don't tell you that you'll be able to survive without much sleep because the simple act of looking at your baby is stirring, gratifying, energizing.

"Can you believe this is our daughter?" I asked Rob for the umpteenth time. He shook his head and we laughed like a pair of mischief-making campers who had gotten away with something. The wonder didn't wear off.

The trick to happy parenthood, we were beginning to believe, was for us to relax. To start being able to enjoy Elizabeth without worrying so much about her survival. To stop expecting our own lives to simply pick up where they'd left off.

Easier said than done. Especially on shattered sleep.

My ob/gyn said I was healing well and assured me that the pouchiness above my incision would soon tighten and the rigidity of my scar would soon soften. "Next time," Dr. Romoff said, "I want to catch the baby and I want Rob to cut the cord, okay?"

"Fine, but it's not going to happen *tout de suite.*"

I mentioned that my books said to feed babies every four hours but that our three-week-old seemed to get hungry every two or three.

"Shh! That's one of the well-kept secrets of parenthood. If people knew how hungry babies get, they'd stop having them. I'd be out of business."

At home Rob was at the changing table. "Elizabeth, Elizabeth, we love you to death," I heard him say. Then he paused. "Well, almost to death." I recalled the morbid words of "Rock-a-Bye Baby": ". . . When the bough breaks, the cradle will fall, and down will come baby, cradle and all."

"How's everything?" I asked.

"Fine. She just took a colossal dump. The French's mustard variety. Do we know anyone with a constipated baby? The cure is putting on a fresh diaper. I've changed her three times since you left."

"One good turd deserves another?" I offered, but Rob looked unamused. "Let's just count our blessings she's a girl. If she were a boy, she'd also be spraying all over us."

I counted our blessings a lot. Though Rob and I were both wiped out, Elizabeth wasn't colicky; she was breaking us into parenthood fairly gently. It amazed me that she often just hung out, eyes open, mouth closed. Somehow I'd thought newborns always slept or wept.

"Enjoy it now," my pediatrician had said. "Peak fussiness occurs between six and eight weeks."

Nights were still long and mornings came too early. One day I awoke at 6:00 A.M. in a panic. "Where's Elizabeth?" I said and sent Rob, equally panicked, equally asleep, flying into her room. He peered into her crib, where she was, as they say, sleeping like a baby, and offering us, for once, a much-needed break.

At seven-thirty I called to Rob from Elizabeth's room. She'd finished nursing and I was trying to pull her off me, but she was the dog and I was the bone. I couldn't break her suction and had started to cry. Rob stuck a fingertip in the corner of her mouth and she let go, then also started to wail.

"How'd I get two crying women in my house?" he asked.

"They don't do dishes, they don't do laundry, and they cry first thing in the morning."

Pretty soon I was clutching my abdomen. "Stop," I pleaded. "It only hurts when I laugh."

Despite occasional setbacks, breast-feeding was going better. At each feeding I'd write down what time it was and which breast I'd started on, and by day's end, I'd once again have proof positive that motherhood is a full-time job. 11:30 R, 2:00 L, 4:30 R, 6:30 L, 9:00 R, 11:00 L, 2:00 R, 5:30 L, 8:00 R, 11:30 L. . . . My daughter cleaved unto me about ten times a day, about half an hour each time. That was about five hours of every twenty-four. We're talking a lot of cleaving.

Lucky babies. So demanding, so well loved. Is that why God made them painfully cute? So parents wouldn't pitch them out the window when the going got rough?

When we needed milk or formula or cat food, Rob usually did the hunting and gathering. Why? Because I didn't mind the Great Indoors. And because I was always on a tight schedule.

The ticking of the proverbial baby clock doesn't stop at childbirth. It picks up speed. If I breast-fed Elizabeth and left the house at noon, by two o'clock she might be hungry again — or I might lactate.

When I was big, passersby knew I was pregnant. Now that I was small, nobody knew I was in a hurry to get home. A few weeks ago, strangers at Zabar's could tell I was about to have a baby, and sometimes offered me their place in line. Now no one knew I'd just had a baby, and that she might need me.

Not that a bottle of formula, which we dubbed "sleep juice," wouldn't do the job. But there was nothing more depressing than rushing home with full breasts only to learn that your child had just been fed and was now sound asleep. I hated pumping.

I suppose we were fortunate that Elizabeth accepted bottles.

I may have been her favorite food source, but one morning she bumped against our friend Ed's arm in a sorry attempt to spring milk. He seemed charmed but passed her back, saying, "Here, better take her before she gives me hickeys."

Ed and Beth, Miguel and Susan, Seth and Lucie, and other friends were great about stopping by, sometimes even with fruit or bagels. Others hadn't called until now and seemed guilty and apologetic about it. I didn't mind. I figured some people were showing their thoughtfulness by calling; others by not calling. The only people I didn't appreciate were the ones who, after inquiring as to Elizabeth's health and ours, blithely asked, "So what else is new?"

Elizabeth slept on our table in her KangaRockaRoo — her plastic yellow La-Z-Boy — while Rob and I ate dinner. We watched her the way some couples watch T.V. Sometimes she seemed inexplicably sad and her lower lip would quiver. Sometimes she got startled and her hands would fly out. And often she seemed content and relaxed, and her body would be peaceful and still. She scarcely moved when she slept, although her mouth would sometimes pucker, as though she were suckling in her dreams.

"Someday she'll come padding in wearing Dr. Dentons and asking for another story," I said.

"Or a glass of water."

"Or help on her homework."

"Or permission to stay up and watch a movie."

"Or permission to go out and watch a movie."

"Or borrow the car keys."

"Or go to the prom."

We looked at her cherubic face.

"She's growing up too fast," we said, almost in unison.

My brothers and sister-in-law, Mark, Eric, and Cynthia, came to spend a week with us. Elizabeth was beginning to focus her eyes and I loved watching everybody get acquainted. They seemed to enjoy her antics: her indelicate yawning, luxurious stretching, unselfconscious burping. Funny that the things she'd soon learn not to do in public were the things she now did best.

We were still waiting for her first heartbreaking smile. I looked up "smile" in Dr. Spock and found that we'd have to be patient for several more weeks. I'd waited thirty-one years for Elizabeth. I could wait a few more weeks for her first gummy grin. Now when she turned up the corners of her mouth, it was usually because she was about to fill her diaper.

"Poor little thing!" Eric said, when suddenly Elizabeth trembled and frowned. "When some kids cry, you want to shut 'em up. When Elizabeth cries, you want to comfort her." Ah, the pull of blood. If Eric and Cynthia ever had a baby, I'd love it with abandon, too.

They had been married ten years and knew — because I kept telling them — that I hoped they'd start trying to conceive. Sure, it was their decision, but I couldn't help putting in my kid-sister two cents.

At one point we all sat down to watch our home video. It began with me nine months pregnant addressing the camera and saying I was "looking forward to childbirth — well, child anyway." Next came hospital shots: first I was big and eager, then yellow and drugged, with Rob at my side in the role of cub reporter. "How do you feel?" "Happy about Elizabeth but not too good." "In pain?" "In discomfort. Let's not dwell on this." Then came scenes of Rob doting wildly as Elizabeth sneezed, hiccuped, and slept. Next were takes of me in mother mode: nursing in the rocker, nursing with the cat, nursing to music. Finally came clips of our friends meeting our daughter.

Because Rob works in the film industry, he is wonderful at making and editing movies. If little Elizabeth didn't convince Eric and Cynthia that babies were worth it, I reasoned, maybe our footage would. I watched them laughing, and hoped the video was having the desired effect. Was it?

We finished the last of the popcorn and flipped the lights back on. Eric sat back, looked at us, and announced, "That was great. It really makes you want to have a" — I held my breath — "camcorder."

Going out to restaurants and staying up late was taking its toll. At one point, Cynthia, who had been very helpful with Elizabeth, said, "The baby is crying."

"So is the mommy," I pointed out and pulled up my shirt.

When Rob and I were short on sleep, he snapped and I sniffled. We knew we needed to take naps.

But my mother knew we also needed a night out by ourselves.

And she made it easy for us: she bought theater tickets and volunteered to baby-sit.

On Elizabeth's four-week birthday, we left her behind for the first time. I wrote Mom a huge list of instructions and phone numbers and succeeded in making us all even more nervous. Then we saw *Driving Miss Daisy*. A perfect choice: an engrossing play with no intermission.

When it ended, we bolted. When a taxi slowed down, we jumped in, blue-haired ladies be damned. On the way home we didn't discuss Morgan Freeman's performance; we discussed Elizabeth. We also realized how wise it was of my mother not to have sent us to a restaurant — we probably would have telephoned between courses and headed home before dessert.

With my whole family in town, Mom and Lewis gave a party in honor of the newest member of the clan.

"Welcome to the rest of your life," said one family friend.

"We knew you had it in you," said another.

Meredith's sister, who has two sons, told me about her invaluable weekly meetings with new mothers.

"Really?" I asked. "I saw a notice in my pediatrician's office about a mother's group. But I didn't know if I'd like the women."

"Carol," she explained, slightly exasperated, "If they're willing to talk about the color of your baby's shit, it doesn't matter if you like them."

Rob carried Elizabeth around in her Snugli. One cousin said she looked just like me; another said she favored Rob. One friend said she resembled my mother; another said she was the image of Rob's mother. It occurred to me that if I didn't love Gene, that could be a nightmare. Imagine how some women might feel having to nurse their mother-in-law in miniature.

Finally there was a man I'd never met who asked, "What do you do?"

"Breast-feed," I was tempted to answer. Instead I told him I was a writer and that I used to be my own boss. "But those days are gone. Now Little One here calls all the shots."

When Elizabeth turned one month old, Rob said, "Now that the move and the holidays are over, I guess my paternity leave is, too." I knew he wanted to get back to work. He'd developed cabin fever and a classic case of provider panic. Lately he'd taken to saying things like, "I can't believe how much diapers cost," and "All we three do is eat," and "Look at these bills! And neither of us is earning any money!"

We had been writing huge checks left and right. Most bills were covered by insurance, but our policy didn't include well-baby care. And the extra days Elizabeth spent at Lenox Hill were because *I* was recuperating, not because *she* was ill. I called the hospital, but rules were rules, and her bill alone cost us over one thousand out-of-pocket dollars.

So Rob went back to work, and I started in on the dishes and laundry. I couldn't complain. I was no longer pregnant or post-op. And I liked knowing I could make it through the day without help. When Elizabeth was asleep, I even managed to answer teen mail and start an article. When she was awake, I put her in the Snugli and went on errands. I'd finally realized that I didn't have to stay indoors until someone could cover for me.

Yet I still couldn't wait for Rob to return each night. I used not to mind when he worked late. I'd write or read, watch T.V., or yak on the phone. Now I started sending out Rob-come-home vibes at five o'clock. Not because I was starved for adult conversation, but because I'd be impatient to toss the baby at him, say, "Your turn!" and run — alone — into the shower or my office.

Usually Rob would appear around seven, as eager to see Elizabeth as I was for him to take over. She was wakeful, he was fresh, and their brief "quality time" seemed so joyous that I'd sometimes wonder, senselessly, if she'd love him more than me. If she'd find me less fun because I spent more time feeding, washing, and changing her, than I did playing with her. It always seemed that she met his eyes more than she met mine.

Of course there were nights when Rob wanted to come home to a mug of beer and a moment of quiet before facing wife, child, and responsibility. Then we'd sometimes argue before we'd even said hello. Though often not. Who had the energy to argue?

Elizabeth was helping us mellow out, ease up. She was putting our world into perspective. A check of mine bounced, and I didn't flinch. Rob broke a wedding-present vase, and we cheerfully swept it up. We had a healthy baby — who cared about nuisances and knickknacks?

Then the biggie: our car got stolen. We'd lent our seven-year-old Honda to a friend and he'd parked it on the park side of Riverside Drive. It was gone by morning. The friend was beside himself. He contacted the pound and the police, and Rob called our insurance agent.

But to everybody's surprise, we remained the picture of calm. How upset can you get when your baby is napping angelically in her KangaRockaRoo?

The theft of our car was a drag, not a tragedy. And we had Elizabeth to thank for teaching us the difference.

Phil, a doorman of our building, insisted I meet Leslie, a woman in 14B. Phil was a born matchmaker and Leslie's baby was just five days younger than mine.

Moments later she and I were sitting side by side on her sofa breast-feeding. It felt like a tribal initiation ritual.

Leslie, twenty-eight, said she used to be a manager on Wall Street but was enjoying the peacefulness of staying at home: "Being with Adam gives me more satisfaction than work ever did."

I was struck by the abrupt and total change in her life. She went from office managing to at-home mommying. We both had adjusting to do, but my switch was more subtle. I was trying to go from writing at home to a combination of mommying and writing at home.

"How did you manage to cut her nails?" Leslie asked.

"I bit them when she was asleep," I admitted. "I knew what I was doing — I've had years of practice."

"How are you coming along on your thank-yous?" I asked.

"I have about sixty to go. Most of my gifts are from groups. I have to write four letters for every teddy bear."

We continued comparing notes. She still hadn't used her baby carrier; I hadn't tried our baby carriage. She felt guilty when she left Adam sleeping and went down the elevator to get the mail; I felt guilty when Elizabeth fussed and I inserted her pacifier rather than rocking her. And neither of us had enough energy for sex even though we were about to get the go-ahead from our ob/gyns.

We agreed to take a walk on the next sunny morning and to start an occasional evening exchange. I'd watch both kids one night; she'd mind them another. Sounded great. I thought of the parenting magazines that had promised me a new circle of buddies. And I almost told Leslie what Rick told Louis in *Casablanca*: "I think this is the beginning of a beautiful friendship."

161

A few days later it was pouring and I had to dash out for a few things. I decided to call Leslie and got her husband, a musician who worked at home. "May I drop Elizabeth off for an hour?" I asked.

"Sure."

"When would be a good time?"

"Anytime is good. Just make sure she's sleepy."

I did, she was, and I ran my errands in record time. I returned, breathless, to find Elizabeth just waking up.

At this stage, baby-sitting really was baby-sitting. Soon enough it would be baby reading, baby feeding, baby changing, baby chasing.

The next night Rob and I dropped Elizabeth off for the evening. This would be our second date without her, our first movie in months. As we headed down the elevator, Rob said, "Do you believe we're leaving our baby with virtual strangers?"

"They're not strangers. We talked for two hours the other day and they've already watched Elizabeth once. Besides, they're 'newborn' parents, too. We even use the same pediatricians."

"You're right," Rob said. "And I trust Laura's instincts."

I looked at him. "Leslie's."

We rode the rest of the way in silence.

I was supposed to baby-sit for Adam, but Leslie canceled. She said he was "colicky" and "impossible" and that they "wouldn't wish him on their worst enemy." The next night, Rob was still at work when Leslie wheeled him in. "You got the raw end of the deal," she said. "Adam's louder."

At first, both well-fed kids gave their pacifiers a workout. Then both hiccuped. Then both dozed. Then both began to howl. I cuddled them, bounced them, quieted them. Elizabeth drifted off to sleep. But no matter how much I patted or sang to Adam, I could only get him to shut his eyes for fifteen-minute stretches. Even asleep, his fists stayed clenched. Though younger than Elizabeth, he was stronger. A bruiser. A boy. A male being programmed, according to mothers of toddlers, to fall under the spell of fire trucks, bulldozers, and freight trains.

By the time Rob showed up, both kids were crying again. How did parents of twins manage? "Feed them!" Rob commanded, but I didn't want to make Leslie pump. "She'll be back in a minute," I said. Besides, I had learned something: crying babies could be held off. I quieted them again by singing and rolling their carriages back and forth. Food, the easy way out, was not the only answer.

Doorman Phil directed Ashley, another new mother in our building, to my door. We sat on my sofa and ate yogurt. A ballet dancer, she said she was enjoying these weeks at home but missed conversation. "I'm used to being virtually naked with people all day. It's hard to get used to privacy."

I was used to privacy. But we did share a frustration. Unlike the working woman who could take a maternity leave — sometimes even paid, no less — and leave her job behind, Ashley and I couldn't really stop. She was anxious to get back into shape. And I was unable (afraid?) to keep my pen capped for three months. I needed to write (if only in my journal).

Carol and Leslie and Ashley. Our building was going through its own private baby boom, and I hoped it could provide the kind of informal mothers' group that people said was so valuable. According to Phil, Elizabeth was now the oldest of five babies under one large roof. And pregnant women were everywhere. "This building used to seem like a nursing home," a neighbor said. "Now it's becoming a nursery!"

We took Elizabeth to Beth and Ed's Third Annual Waffle Fest. She slept three hours straight, and since everybody claimed they wanted to hold her, she was passed around like a bowl of chips.

At four she woke up hungry. I lifted my sweater discreetly, but Rob announced, "Elizabeth's favorite song is 'Thanks for the Mammaries.'"

Back home an enormous package was waiting from his aunt. "Finally!" I said. Rob assembled the swing she had promised us, but complained that it was surburban-sized.

"Oh, c'mon, this is a godsend."

"God did not send this," he replied, distressed that his neat-and-tidy home was being slowly taken over by baby paraphernalia. Maybe He didn't. But I knew how handy the swing would be. I knew because Leslie had one.

Rob and I were glad our eight-pound, five-week-old daughter was such a napper. Glad she was "easy" and "good." But now we had a new worry: was she a bore? She got a ten for looks, but what about personality? Did she have any zest? Any joie de vivre?

"Is she a blob? At times a cross-eyed blob?" I asked.

"On personality, I'm afraid she might be a four," Rob lamented.

I'd just shown him a card from a college friend, Hilary, whose baby girl was born two days before Elizabeth. It read: "Kate is a wondrous, eager little person who has us absolutely captivated. I literally could sit and look at her all day."

I glanced at Elizabeth. She was out cold.

"If she's a blob," Rob said, "at least she's our blob." He squeezed her toes.

I wasn't done fretting. Maybe *I* was the blob. Was I stimulating her enough when she was awake? Should I be flashing pictures in front of her in black, white, and primary colors?

"Give the kid a break," my high-school friend Judy coached on the phone from Minneapolis. "The world is stimulating enough. You like parties, but it's nice when the guests go home, right? Newborn babies need lots of quiet."

I felt reassured. Sort of. But when I ran into my friend Nancy and her new baby, now three months old, and when I saw how tuned in he was, I confessed that Elizabeth was still kind of zoned out. "C'mon, Harry was clueless until a few weeks ago," Nancy said. "Elizabeth will be alert and responsive in no time. You'll see. Rob will be dragging her off to Yankees games."

I must have looked skeptical.

"Listen," Nancy continued. "Mothers always worry about whether they're feeding their children too little or too much, holding them too little or too much, stimulating them too little or too much. You know what? Kids all grow up."

A nice insight, but that night Elizabeth wouldn't take my breast or her pacifier. She felt hot and I felt helpless. And the more I worried about her, the tighter I hugged her, the more I loved her.

The next morning, instead of lunging at me and going at it like a vacuum cleaner, she suckled poorly then conked out. I'd never seen a creature sleep so much — with the possible exception of my cat. New mothers talk about how sleepy they are, but not how sleepy their babies are. Elizabeth left me engorged as well as distressed. I called the doctor and he said to bring her in if she didn't perk up by the afternoon.

I did. "I know you gave her a clean bill of health just a few days ago," I said, "but would you mind checking her again? I'm probably being paranoid, but she seems so listless."

Naturally Elizabeth chose that moment to wake up, eat voraciously, and soil not one, not two, but three of the blue paper pads they put out for babies to lie on.

"I guess she's come around," I said sheepishly. Why had I hauled her back to the pediatrician? Why hadn't I interpreted her sleepiness as a generous gift, a lovely grace period, a "Hey, Ma, you've been through a lot. Why don't you rest up?"

Dr. Kahn allowed as to how she may have had a little bug, and, after poking and probing, said she looked fine. "Don't worry about minor fluctuations," he said, "but if she ever has a high fever or seems off for twenty-four hours, let us know."

I went home relieved and decided not to let myself feel stupid. Elizabeth's health was important. So was my peace of mind.

Ringo Starr came on the radio and Elizabeth and I danced along. "You're six weeks, you're beautiful, and you're mine," I crooned, taking poetic license.

We'd come a long way in a short time. When she was awake, she now looked instead of merely seeing. She even engaged us in wondrous staredowns. She still hadn't flashed us her pearly gums, but some of her newborn clothes were getting snug — and some of my pants were beginning to zip up. And now when she slept on the KangaRockaRoo in the middle of the dining-room table, I felt it was okay to let her out of my sight for a quick moment, to seize the opportunity to take a shower, make a call, haul out the trash.

Rob wanted to go out to celebrate her six-week birthday.

"I don't know," I said. "At home when she cries, I worry about her. At a restaurant when she cries, I worry about everybody."

"She'll be good," he insisted.

I hesitated.

"Carol," he said, "when we eat in, I do all the cooking and cleaning."

"Most of it," I corrected and got my coat and Elizabeth's baby bag. I used to feel guilty about our domestic inequity. Rob spent a lot more time in the kitchen than I did. But he enjoyed it more than I did. And it was fast becoming clear that I'd be spending much more time in the nursery.

Lisa and Andy arrived from Boston with our niece, Sarah, Rob's sister Sally, and her boyfriend, Aden.

"So has it been hell?" Aden asked, getting right to the point.

"No, it's been great," I said, but was overcome by a yawn. "I could do with a little uninterrupted sleep."

"Your nails are polished," Lisa observed. "You must have things under control."

"Don't be fooled. It's only the second time since Elizabeth's birth."

After dinner Andy said, "I've never seen such an energetic baby. Can you believe how many hours she's been up?"

I was awash with gratitude. My baby: energetic.

Sally said she dreamed she was going to baby-sit Elizabeth, but when she picked her up, she was astonished at how heavy she was. Freud could dine out on that one, I thought. Sally also asked to see my baby pictures, and I showed her the few I have. Being the third kid of a working mother made for a pretty slim scrapbook. "She looks exactly like you," Sally said, and though Elizabeth had bald spots and a rapidly receding hairline, I swelled with pride.

Clearly, my in-laws were the perfect guests. Though the corners of Elizabeth's lips still wouldn't budge, our visitors doted on her endlessly. Rob and I lapped it up.

At bedtime, we tucked her in her carrier crib and put our niece in Elizabeth's crib. Then we peered in to steal a glimpse of the future. Sarah weighed only fifteen pounds but looked enormous.

"I'm not ready for Bitsy to get so big," I whispered.

"I'm not either," Rob said. "Little Lizard."

One reason we'd named our daughter Elizabeth was because it was such a stately name. Heaven forbid anyone should call her Betty, Beth, Liz, or Lib in our presence. Yet we were guilty of calling her every name in the book, from Bitsy and Lizard to Pee Wee and Cubby. I hoped we'd quit before she started talking.

"Isn't it nice having a baby?" I said, facing Rob in bed.

"You want to have another one?" he asked.

"Not yet."

"Maybe we should before Elizabeth realizes what's going on and before we realize how much work is really involved."

"Rob, I'm nowhere near ready."

There was a pause.

"So are we allowed?"

Another pause.

"I was hoping you wouldn't ask."

"When did it happen?"

"A few days ago."

"I missed it?"

"You missed it."

"Well how about tonight?"

"We don't have condoms and I haven't been refitted for a diaphragm and I'm tired and sore and I've been suckled and cuddled all day."

"I take it that's a no?"

"It's a 'Soon.'"

Unfortunately, now that we had a baby, I wasn't the least bit randy. Maybe God really did make sex for procreation. I remembered the old cigarette ad, "I'd rather fight than switch," and thought, I'd rather sleep than screw.

But Rob liked my big breasts and small waist. He complained that once again the gods had given him a sex toy — batteries not included.

Chanda was eighteen years old. Elizabeth was seven weeks. I left them both with Rob and went to see Dr. Romoff.

"When I was pregnant, I got this little spot on my face and it's still there. Is that okay?"

"Perfectly normal. It's a freckle."

"When I breast-feed, a little bubble of milk always forms on the areola above my right nipple. Is that okay?"

"Perfectly normal. It's an accessory duct."

He checked me over and declared me healthy. I was six pounds heavier than I was before I got pregnant, but my diaphragm size was actually smaller. He prescribed a new one, then issued official permission: Rob and I could have intercourse again.

Lord, help me.

The mail brought this letter:

> I am thirteen years old and I really like a guy and he's sixteen. If I went out with him, do you think he'd expect me to "do stuff"? Also, is there a difference between making love and sex? Also, it seems that sex is always on my mind! Also, if I do go out with this guy, do you think it's a wise idea to go over while his parents aren't home? He lives across the street. I'd appreciate it if you could answer me really soon.
>
> P.S. Are you going to write another book? If you do, could you do it about older guys and sex?

I got out my pen and thought, Lord, help us all.

That night as I fed Elizabeth and tucked her in, Rob lit candles all around our room.

"Hi," he said when I came in.

"Hi." He took off my shirt. "Wait, hang on. Slow down. Ouch! I told you not to kiss my breasts."

"I know. I'm sorry. But you can't blame me for being attracted to them. *She's* attracted to them."

"Tell me about it." I picked up my notepad, stalling for time. "In the last twenty-four hours, I've nursed her at midnight, three, six, eight, ten, noon, three, six, eight, and eleven."

"I can't believe I married a woman who takes notes on everything," he said. "And just because the baby gets you all the time doesn't mean I shouldn't get you at all." He caressed my shoulders.

"I know." I kissed him. We got in bed. But I still felt like a nervous virgin. What if I lactated during sex? Would there be two wet spots? Three? I considered suggesting we stop and have a few drinks. I could do that, couldn't I? Elizabeth wasn't driving anywhere.

But it was too late. "Rob, this hurts!"

"I'm sorry. I'll be gentle."

"Ouch, ouch, ouch. Wait, wait, wait."

"Should I stop?"

"No. I don't know. We should probably just do it." My eyes were wet. "I had no idea it was going to hurt."

"I'll be gentle."

"Okay. Wait! Don't thrust." Poor guy hadn't thrust in ages.

"Why am I so sore?" I asked. Had I once read something about breast-feeding and dryness? Maybe the real reason women rarely conceive while nursing is because they rarely have sex while nursing.

We finished what we started: we consummated our parenthood.

But barely, just barely.

At 3:00 A.M. Elizabeth got me up. I fed her while flipping through my pregnancy and childbirth books. There it was: dyspareunia, painful sex.

In the morning I called the ob/gyn.

"May I say what this is regarding?" asked the receptionist.

"Dyspareunia," I said. Discretion was my middle name.

"It hurt," I told Dr. Romoff. "I thought I'd be spared. I thought that'd be the one advantage of having had a C-section."

"Your hormones and muscles are out of whack," he said. "Be patient. Use a lubricant. It'll take a few weeks."

A few weeks? It might take that long before I was willing to try again.

I needed a phone hug.

I called two close friends, one single, one married. The single woman said, "It's not because of your seven-week hiatus. I've gone much longer and I'm here to say it doesn't hurt when you start again." The married woman said her ob/gyn gave her such a good episiotomy after the birth of their second child that sex was better than ever. "We considered writing him a thank-you note."

So much for moral support.

Several nights later Rob and I gave it another try. It hurt a little less. It felt a little better.

But we still had a long way to go.

I thought I'd be quickly bored and frustrated. I wasn't. I was in love. I'd made the decision to cut back on my work because I realized this was an important time in Elizabeth's development. I hadn't realized it was an important time in mine, too. I'd counted on making sacrifices for Elizabeth. I hadn't counted on her giving back so much, on her winning me over so completely.

Not only was she teaching me to take stock and to streamline my life, but I liked when her eyes lit up. I liked watching her watch me with her steady unblinking gaze. I liked how in seconds she could go from sad to happy, and how even from behind the pacifier, her face could suddenly look expectant and gleeful. I liked dressing and undressing her (she was a clotheshorse already). And I liked her smile.

Her smile. At first it was a fleeting, tentative half smile, directed sometimes at us, sometimes at the wall. Even then we found it so endearing we could hardly bear it — a baby's smile must open the last floodgates of a parent's love. When her smile became more real, more deliberate, we were beside ourselves. We even loved what her smile was not: it was not self-conscious or manipulative or camera-ready. It was a gift, no strings attached.

One night, when everyone was sleeping except 7-Eleven clerks, disc jockeys, frazzled lawyers, and nursing mothers, Elizabeth began to cry. I was beat, disoriented. But I swung my feet to the floor and staggered to her room.

She greeted me with a grin worth waking for. She appreciated my coming, and that was all I asked. Someday I might be harder to please. Someday she might be harder to please. For now, we were all each other wanted.

I looked out the window and noticed rectangles of light in the dark buildings nearby. Were other mothers and babies eyeing each other sleepily, lovingly? During midnight feedings, I sometimes closed my eyes, sometimes breezed through novels. Often I'd notice the clock and think, "Gee, I should call Europe or something." Other times I just studied Elizabeth and pondered the chain of mothers and daughters and mothers and daughters who came before and would come after us.

Breast-feeding continued to fill me with conflicting emotions. On the one hand, it was exhausting to be Elizabeth's personal food processor. I yearned for a day off, for an uninterrupted night's sleep. There were times when I looked down at my frantically nursing child and thought of Paul McCartney's words: "Do you love me like you know you ought to do? . . . Or is this the only thing you want me for?"

On the other hand, I reveled in it. I was already sad that I'd have to wean in time for my book tour. When my baby turned four months old, my book would be in the stores, and I'd be on the road. Still a long way off, but would I be ready?

At times I felt sorry that Rob was missing out. Sure, he could spend long days in the world and long nights in bed, but he couldn't feel what I felt.

There was something so unutterably sweet about Elizabeth's tender tugging, her unabashed animal noises. When she held on to my bra, I was charmed. When she wailed desperately — turning red, scarcely inhaling — I loved knowing I could quiet her in seconds. I enjoyed feeling so needed, being the proud provider.

Sometimes she'd be so ravenous that when I switched her from one breast to the other, she'd burst into tears of outrage. "Oh, ye of little faith," I'd say. Sometimes she'd grunt as I rearranged her in my arms, straightened her folded ear, squeezed her now-chubby thighs. When she was done, her head would flop, her body slump, and she'd look drunk and satisfied.

Such was the power of my bosom.

I popped Elizabeth in her Snugli and zipped up a jacket I'd borrowed from Rob. As I walked, her feet tapped my belly. It reminded me of when I carried her inside me. But now when I sang to her, it looked as though I were talking to myself.

"What'cha got in there?" asked a construction worker.

"A baby." I unzipped the jacket just enough to reveal her sleepy face and the pink pom-pom of her hat.

"Congratulations!"

"Thanks!"

I picked up photos (we still hadn't caught her smile on film). I bought a black miniskirt (I couldn't wait to look chic again). And I went to a health food store to buy some fresh-ground peanut butter.

"Your shoelace is untied," said the man behind the counter.

"I know." I'd been trying to figure out how to bend with the Snugli on. Where was Rob when I needed him?

"Can I tie it for you?"

"I'd appreciate it."

And they say New Yorkers aren't friendly.

Extra! Extra! An attractive man made a pass at me. "You have beautiful eyes. Why are you walking so fast?"

I was taken aback. "Because I'm rushing home to be with my baby." I whipped out her photo. "Now *she* has beautiful eyes," I said.

We were waiting for the crosswalk light to turn. I commented on his accent and asked where he was from.

Argentina.

He said he ran a travel agency and asked if I'd like to have a cup of coffee.

"No, but I have some lovely friends who might." In Manhattan, you hate to let a good-looking heterosexual get away.

"You mean like a blind date?"

"Something like that."

"I can't," he said. "I'm married."

Rob said we should start in on our taxes. Taxes? Wasn't it still Christmas? I remembered when Dad died on April 7, six years earlier, and how surprised I was that the world kept turning. That summer came anyway.

Birth, like death, makes you lose track of time. In my mind, it wasn't February, it was December. I knew the days were ticking by. I knew I'd soon be saying Elizabeth's age in months instead of weeks. I was already forgetting to honor every Thursday, her birth day. But it was hard to believe that parenthood was growing on us. That we were beyond consulting Spock three times daily. Beyond forcing our guests to look at all our photos and videos.

I applied for a social security number for Elizabeth. In response to "Relationship to the applicant," I wrote, "Mother." Me, a mom. Forms always make things hit home. I remembered when I first had to check "deceased" after "Father" on a medical report.

Still, it couldn't be time to think about taxes. Not yet. The notion made me weak with fatigue.

But then, everything did. Despite my moments of rapture, I was spent, played out. And overjoyed when Rob came home — home for another whole weekend.

He looked at Elizabeth with amazement. "Look how she turns her head! And listen to her little baby noises! She's trying so hard to talk." On cue Elizabeth started to hum, mew, and coo, to make baby sounds and baby songs.

Rob picked her up and danced her around the room singing, "I'm in love with a wonderful girl!"

Though I didn't feel jealous (would I ever?), I interjected, "How about me?"

"I'm in love with you, too," he said, giving me a hand so we could all three sway to the music.

Our marriage was changing. Instead of going to movies and

restaurants, we were renting videos and ordering in. Instead of having sex, we were having milk shakes. But we now had more in common than ever: we shared a living, breathing child whom we both adored with a bonding passion.

On weekends I'd plan to take time for myself, but it was hard. I enjoyed watching Rob with Elizabeth. I enjoyed being with my family.

Rob called from the bathtub where he was floating our daughter on the giant sponge. "Is she getting uglier?" he asked.

"Rob!"

"You know how people say babies look like Winston Churchill?"

"Yeah."

"Does ours look like Buddy Hackett?"

I leaned in for a closer look. "Kinda."

"Everyone used to say how beautiful she was."

"I know. They went into a whole song and dance about how lots of babies aren't cute but you have to pretend they are, but that ours really is."

"And now?"

"Now they cough and sputter and can't help but notice that she's double-chinned and nearly bald."

"You think she peaked at four weeks?"

"Nope."

"Me neither."

On Valentine's Day I was scheduled to be a guest on a radio show about love. I was supposed to go on from 11:00 P.M. to 2:00 A.M. with the hosts, a married couple. I'd done radio and T.V. before, but this time I felt nervous. My plan was to nurse Elizabeth before and after, and I wondered, for starters, if I'd be able to stay awake and animated during the hours on the air.

The answer: yes. When listeners learned I was a Dear Abby type, the phones started ringing. A father called because his eleven-year-old daughter was head over heels about a rock star. A thirteen-year-old called because the boy she liked liked someone else. A seventeen-year-old called because she was in love with two guys.

When we signed off, the hosts and producer said they'd never gotten so many calls and that they'd have me back.

At home I woke Elizabeth and nursed her. "Mommy's in a good mood," I whispered. "Tonight she officially started juggling." I was a radio guest one minute, a mom the next. And I hadn't dropped the ball.

"Catch!" the instructor called, but I missed, and that ball went flying down the hall. Why had I let Nancy talk me into this postpartum exercise class? On the mat, a dozen out-of-shape moms pointed, flexed, stretched, reached, pressed, bent, threw, caught, inhaled, exhaled, and sweat. I couldn't believe I'd paid money for this torture and humiliation — or that I'd done aerobics three times a week in my misspent youth.

"I don't know if I'm coming back," I said to Nancy as we went to the baby-care room to retrieve Harry and Elizabeth.

We heard a cacophony of cries, but Elizabeth looked merry. "She has such a sweet disposition," said the sitter. "She smiled and looked interested the whole time and just now fell asleep."

I beamed and made a note to relay this report card to both grandmothers.

"Well *I'm* coming back," Nancy said. "Every other day this month."

"You're earnest."

"I'm desperate."

At brunch at Leslie's, every couple had a baby and a story. One woman said, almost boastfully, that her labor "was the most horrible, awful pain, but when it was over, it was over. It stopped the second the baby was born."

"That's when mine started," I said. "I had a C-section. Elizabeth was jack-knifed inside me, fanny down."

"Now that I'm not worried about stillbirth," another woman admitted, "I'm worried about crib death."

"What's your biggest worry?" Leslie asked me.

"The DPT shot," I answered.

Cut to: The Doctor's Office, DPT Day.

Elizabeth snuggled innocently in my arms, unaware of the betrayal that lay ahead. The nurse put her on the scale. "Ten pounds four ounces. Twenty-two inches." She moved Elizabeth back to the examining table. "C'mon, Chunky," she said.

Chunky? My kid? Maybe it was time to cut out the milk shakes.

Dr. Kahn studied Elizabeth's weight and length chart. (Infants are measured in length, not height.)

"How's she measure up?" I asked, stalling for time.

"Fiftieth percentile for both. You're looking at an average-sized two-month-old." I thought of Gloria Steinem's line, "This is what fifty looks like." And I wondered if Elizabeth might someday tower over her petite mom.

"The DPT immunization protects against diphtheria, pertussis (whooping cough), and tetanus," the doctor said. "She'll need booster shots at four and six months."

My eyes filled with tears. I hoped he didn't notice.

"The benefits outweigh the risks, but no medicine is without risk. About fifty percent of babies react badly and become

181

cranky after the shot." He gave Elizabeth six milliliters of Panadol, an acetaminophen for babies.

She started to bawl.

"Oh, Sweetie." I hugged her. "He's about to really give you something to cry about."

"I'm afraid I am."

"And what about the greater risks? What happens to babies with extreme reactions?"

"They go into a coma or have convulsions. But that's very, very rare."

My eyes teared up again. How could people tell dead baby jokes?

"Hold her on your lap." He swabbed her thigh. I cringed. "Here we go."

The needle went in. Her mouth flung open. Her face turned red. There was total silence.

Then she cried, louder and longer than ever before.

"Breathe!" I said, only half in jest. "Breathe! Breathe! Breathe!"

She inhaled then screamed again. It was pitiful.

I took her home and, mercifully, she fell asleep. But I kept vigil over her crib. I knew she was alive because the ring of her pacifier bobbed up and down, and her belly was gently rising and falling. Soon I began to feel headachy and feverish myself, and I climbed into my own bed.

Elizabeth slept all day, waking only to feed and cry. When Rob came home at eight-thirty, he found two cranky females, one with a swollen thigh, the other with a swollen breast.

"Why didn't you come home earlier?" I asked.

"I should have called. But I was out making money. And then I stopped to buy us food for dinner." He leaned over, lips puckered, but the kiss was for Elizabeth.

"If I weren't at home with our baby all day I could be making money too, so you're not allowed to lord that over us."

"I'm not lording it over you."

"And I'd rather have just soup with you than wait an hour for a big meal."

Rob sighed. He'd learned not to push when I was being irrational.

Elizabeth, however, burst into tears.

Seemed all three of us had had a hard day.

Susan was due in less than two months. I called to get her list of friends for a baby shower we were hosting. And I told her I was reading about the importance of bonding.

"If a goat is separated from her kid for the first hour after birth, she rejects it forever. If a goose sees a person after birth, it thinks the person is its mother and follows it around. The thing that bums me out is that after my C-section, Elizabeth and I didn't exactly commune. And now it's too late for all those wonderful benefits. But it's not too late for you, so talk to your ob/gyn and bond your heart out."

"Carol, can I tell you something?"

"What?"

"You're not a goat or a goose."

I laughed. I found her observation immensely reassuring.

"So how's it going?" she asked. "Is motherhood what you expected?"

Yes. No. What did I expect — besides a broadening of my hips and horizons?

"Motherhood is moody stuff," I confessed. "I understand Elizabeth better now. I can usually tell if she needs to be put to bed or to my breast, or if she just needs a toy. But every time I think I've got her number, she changes it. And I miss having time to work — and time to fritter away."

Now that people were once again asking, "What do you do?" instead of "When are you due?" I was also beginning to feel that I had to justify myself. "I think having had a 'working mom' messed me up on this one," I told Susan. "I mean, there are days when I am totally busy grocery shopping, doing laundry, and taking care of Elizabeth, but I wind up feeling like I didn't get anything done."

"You're being too hard on yourself."

"I know. It even pains me that our *New York Times* are stacking up. I feel rebuked each morning. I wish we lived in a town with a skinny newspaper."

"No, you don't."

"No, I don't. But I can't catch up. And when I do, the news is full of drowned babies and burned babies. That's my reading. All I'm writing is thank-you notes. And checks."

"You sound like you need a drink."

"It's just lack of sleep. I probably should have half a beer. Did I tell you that when Rob heard beer can help a woman's let-down reflex, he thought that was for women who felt let down that their kids were scrunched-up prune-faces?"

Susan laughed. "What's Elizabeth doing these days?"

"Let me see. When I hold her, she's beginning to hang on, to hold back." The pressure of her fingers on my shoulders was slight and sweet and new. Each hug brought on a rush of motherlove. "And she's become so easy to please. What's fascinating is how everything fascinates her. A pattern, a light, her own fingers. She's taking it all in."

"I can't wait."

I told her to be sure she had all the modern conveniences. A Snugli for carrying the baby. A swing for calming the baby. A microwave for warming bottles. A cordless phone so she could change the baby while gossiping. A remote control so she could change the channel while nursing. A V.C.R. so she and Miguel could still go to the movies.

"V.C.R.? We're your friends in the dark ages, remember? We still use the black-and-white T.V. you guys forced on us years ago."

The one I had as a kid, back when the children on my block were reared on cartoons and candy. Miguel grew up in a house with no T.V., and he and Susan didn't believe in letting their minds go to mush. While we kept up with Hope and Michael, they reread Dostoyevsky. I could only admire them.

I wasn't through offering unsolicited advice. I told her to befriend pregnant neighbors. "This ballet dancer, Ashley, hired this Peruvian woman, Matilde, to baby-sit her six-week-old. Ashley asked if I wanted to drop off Elizabeth two mornings a week. At first I felt too cheap to hire a sitter. Elizabeth is usually napping or nursing. But Ash and I each give Matilde ten dollars and the freedom makes me giddy. It's a small price to pay for a little time off."

"That's great. When did you start?"

"Thursday. On Elizabeth's ten-week birthday. It's day care in my own building. And by noon, I'm that much more psyched to be a mom again."

Susan swore she'd be on the lookout for pregnant ladies in the elevator. "Hey, listen, I have to ask you a favor."

"Shoot."

"My ob/gyn thinks I should wear a maternity girdle for my back pains and I can't find one in Brooklyn Heights. Since you live near Mothercare, could you buy me one — if they have them? Miguel can send a messenger for it and I'll reimburse you."

"No problem." And it wasn't. Except that I bought the wrong size, so Miguel the high-powered lawyer had to send a second messenger to return it to me the next day, and then a third messenger to pick up the right one.

Made me wonder what was inside all the other plain brown packages being rushed around town.

In Spanish, *mama* means mother and *mamar* means to nurse. I was in the rocking chair breast-feeding Elizabeth. She studied me with smiling eyes while clutching my free breast as though to claim it. Ordinarily this might have felt like one of those warm 'n' fuzzy mothering moments.

But I was in possession of a bum bosom, a left breast that wasn't working. Soft underneath, hard on top, it hurt like hell.

I called the ob/gyn. Nurse Liz said to try compresses and massage. "But don't let down your milk and leave it there. That'll just make things worse." She also recommended other nursing positions besides the Madonna technique. "Try lying down. Or the football hold. If you're still sore in the morning, we can give you antibiotics for mastitis."

Mastitis. I looked it up in my Dr. Spock and Dr. Mom books but found only masturbation. Not now, thanks.

I tried massaging and pumping and hot compresses and nursing. My breast got bigger and harder and redder and sorer. No way could I hold out until morning.

I called Stephanie, Rob's cousin. She was both an ob/gyn and a new mother.

"My boob is about to explode," I said. "The top half is engorged to the max."

"Does the nipple have a white spot on it?"

"Yes."

"The size of the head of a pin?"

"Yes!"

"I've had the exact problem. This is what I suggest: you sterilize a needle and prick the tip of the spot."

This didn't sound one bit appealing, but Stephanie was a doctor and I was desperate.

"I sterilize a needle . . . ?"

"Right. Wipe it with alcohol. Then don't jab yourself or any-

187

thing, just burst the blister. I bet an ounce of milk will come shooting out. I bet it will be like a geyser."

I winced, thanked her, and took to the tub, where I gingerly took aim. One prick and I hit pay milk. It was Geyser City, Yellowstone National Park. My breast decompressed, and I pumped enough for a supplementary bottle.

I wrote Stephanie a "You're a genius!" postcard and called Nurse Liz.

"Well, it's a creative solution," she acknowledged. "I'll pass it on to other patients in need."

"That's why I called. To help other mastitic masochists." I almost added, Say that three times fast.

On Elizabeth's eleven-week birthday, she slept from midnight to 6:00 A.M. The six-hour stretch of sleep was a first for both of us, and I hoped we were onto something big.

We weren't. It was a fluke. The next night she got me up at one, four, and six.

At six, she nursed with concentrated effort. When she was done, she looked up, seemed surprised to see me, and gave me an enormous smile. I smiled back, besotted. But I wondered: whose bosom did she think she'd been suckling, anyway?

We were having dinner in the corner of a restaurant with Rob's aunt, uncle, and a few of their friends. I wore an oversize shirt and was sitting next to a long-winded fellow who talked incessantly about his dry-cleaning business. Elizabeth was on my lap having supper.

Over coffee, he paused for breath, and asked how old my baby was. "Are you nursing her?" he inquired next, clearly a question in the abstract.

I looked straight at him. Was this guy for real?

"Even as we speak," I answered.

He turned crimson. I loved it. I felt pleased that I was able to feed Elizabeth so inconspicuously. And though I should have been ashamed of myself, I got a kick out of making him feel foolish.

I'd resisted temptation many times during my pregnancy. When strangers asked, "How many months along are you?" I'd sometimes wanted to answer, "I'm not pregnant, just fat." But I'd never once been a smart-ass.

I figured it was high time.

Debbie, an editor at *Redbook*, asked if I wanted to run their annual Top Ten Children's Picture Books of the Year contest. It involved reading hundreds of new children's books, some administrative coordinating, lining up judges, and writing an article for the Christmas issue. "Will I get to keep some of the books?" I asked, trying not to sound too eager.

"Sure. Lots of them."

I accepted, thrilled.

I figured this was one assignment I'd be able to manage. The books would come, I'd put Elizabeth on my lap, I'd say, "C'mon, kid, we've got a job to do," and I'd get to feel like a professional and a mom all at once.

I still had only six hours a week of child care, but Elizabeth napped a lot, and since I knew my time was so limited, I was usually able to gear up and work more efficiently than ever.

Except, of course, when I was bleary-eyed, spaced-out, and brain-dead. Then it was all I could do to get through the newspaper.

Almost twelve weeks old, Elizabeth was going on her first trip. We were not traveling light. Not only were we taking skis, ski boots, ski poles, ski pants, and other grown-up essentials to Utah, but we were taking Elizabeth's carrier crib, bouncing chair, clothes, blankets, diapers, baby wipes, bottles, pacifiers, and toys. By the time we'd finished packing, we were so exhausted that it was a good thing we were going on vacation.

New parents had told us that it was easier to travel with a baby than a toddler. Maybe so, but I was worried, for starters, about Elizabeth's ears popping.

"Just be sure she's swallowing during takeoff and landing," the pediatrician said. "She needs to be sucking on something. A pacifier, a bottle, your breast. It makes no difference."

No difference? I considered feeling offended. "And if her ears don't pop?"

"Then she'll cry and that will pop them."

The flight was easy and quiet. The flight attendant had us board first ("Parenthood has its privileges," Rob whispered). And when Elizabeth fretted, I fed her. More than necessary, no doubt, but I'm sure our fellow passengers appreciated the quiet.

It was hard to believe that my bony baby was now a roly-poly butterball, a chipmunk-cheeked chowhound. She had thunder thighs, and her arms were so plump, it looked like she had rubber bands on her wrists.

When we met Rob's parents, Gene couldn't get over the change. She seized Elizabeth upon our arrival and barely let go. Ken kept his distance and referred to her as "the kid." He also said that vacationing with children was like third-class travel in Bulgaria. But he was intrigued, we could tell. He told her to "wipe that silly grin" off her face, and she smiled all the more.

It was great vacationing *en famille*. My mother-in-law and I had always gotten along, but now we'd grown closer. Her own daughters sometimes complained that she was overinvolved with their lives, calling too often or worrying too much about their classes or jobs, boyfriends or family. And Rob and I had often teased Gene for talking slowly and for the singsong lilt in her voice — characteristics developed after decades of teaching preschoolers. But now that we had a preschooler of our own, we were able to fully appreciate her expressive nurturing side. Gene held her own at dinner parties, but she shone in a room full of children.

When Gene was on "cub patrol," I loved being able to shower, take walks, and even go skiing without undue uneasiness. And Elizabeth got twice the usual number of hugs and kisses. Was this what it was like to live on a kibbutz or in an extended family? If so, it was ideal for some babies, parents, and grandparents. Later it might feel like too many eyes, arms, and egos, but a few years of intergenerational living at this stage might offer more advantages than disadvantages.

Our routine most days was for me to ski in the morning, for Gene to ski in the afternoon, for Rob to pinch-hit for both of us, and for everybody to meet at lunchtime.

When I skied off at 8:00 A.M., I'd leave my mother-in-law directions and a bottle of breast milk. (Have pump, will travel.) It seemed awfully personal. I didn't mind nursing under wraps in front of my in-laws. But for them to open the refrigerator for a Coors and come across a tucked-away bottle of my yellow-gray milk . . . that embarrassed me.

As I shooshed down the slope each morning, my thoughts would still be with Elizabeth. What were she and Gene doing? Did Gene remember her hat? Her sunscreen? Was Elizabeth feeling jolly, her eyes round, her mouth open? Or was she subdued, her expression quizzical as she quietly observed everything around her? Or was she sad — real tears rolling down her soft pretty face? After a couple of runs, I'd let go, separate, daydream, and revel in the fresh air, white sunshine, and what Utah P.R. people call "the greatest snow on earth."

One day at noon, I reached the summit lodge at the top of the mountain, as planned. I found a sign at the warming hut: "Carol Weston, Baby Is At Base Cafeteria." I didn't panic. I wouldn't be able to ski and panic at the same time. But I did speed down the mountain faster than ever before, all the while berating myself for having been selfish and irresponsible, and hoping — please, God — that nothing was wrong.

Nothing was. Gene said there'd been a wind alert in Park City, and that they wouldn't let the baby ride up the gondola to our prearranged meeting place. So we ate pea soup at the base, I traded my parka for Elizabeth, and I held her extra close all afternoon.

What a difference a year made. When we were at the same condo the previous April, I'd worried about poaching Elizabeth in utero. Now when I emerged from the hot tub, instead of fainting, I held my baby. Last year I'd enjoyed the library just east of the condo. This year I noticed, for the first time, a playground just west. Last year I was finding out that I was pregnant. This year we were making the transition to parenthood. Our lives were being redefined by a living Kewpie doll, a baby with a bald spot who responded to the slightest flirtation with kicks and gurgles and loving looks.

On our last morning in Utah, I pulled Elizabeth into bed to nurse her. Rob woke up and said how cute we looked: a big head and a little head peering out above the covers. "When you move or change jobs, you're not always sure you did the right thing," he said. "But when you have a baby, you know you have. It's what we're for. I feel like we've satisfied a primal urge." He put his arm around me; I put mine around Elizabeth.

At home, one of our favorite games was Baby in the Mirror. I'd hold Elizabeth in front of a mirror and say, "Who's that?" She'd check herself out, look at me, and break into a big smile.

She liked what she saw. So did I.

Our daughter had reached another adorable age. She'd lost some baby fat, grown some hair, and become quite the smiler. She was also learning to sleep, which cheered *me* no end.

If we put her to bed at midnight, she'd often make it until five. I'd long since developed "mother's ears" and got right up when she needed me. But if I gave her a pacifier instead of feeding her, she sometimes gave me two more hours of sleep. The pleasure of climbing back into bed at 5:05 almost made up for the strain of crawling out.

There were other mundane miracles. Her kicks were hardier. Her grasp was stronger. She could hold on to her smallest stuffed animal. (Well, almost. She was hardly rattle-ready.)

And she was talking and vocalizing more and more. Though a long way from "mama" or "dada," she had found her voice and begun to experiment with it. When she was singing, I'd sometimes dial the home number of a working friend who had an answering machine — and let Elizabeth leave a message.

Ashley, my dancer friend, said we seemed to be focusing on Elizabeth's mind while they were working on Eliakim's body.

"What do you mean?"

She pointed out that we often let our three-month-old lie back in her La-Z-Boy while we talked to her, sang to her, read to her, and let her look at dangling objects. They, meanwhile, kept holding up their two-month-old to see if she'd stand and turning her over to see if she'd roll.

I hadn't thought about it.

We were in Ashley's living room with a friend of hers and

her three-and-a-half-month-old son. Right in front of us, for the very first time, the boy rolled over. We mothers were amazed. The boy did it again: threw his legs in the air, flopped them over, followed through with his body. I praised the baby and complimented the mom.

Back home, I tried holding Elizabeth up. She buckled. I tried rolling her on our bed. At first she seemed nonplussed. Then she spat up.

Comparison could be dangerous. It could invite unsavory feelings from smugness to worry. I was glad I was finding like-minded mothers, but I wondered if while yuppies try to keep up with the Joneses, mommies try to keep up with the Joneses' baby.

Elizabeth startled easily and sneezed often. Was that normal? She was fascinated by lights. Was that common? She could amuse herself with a bridge of toys bobbing overhead. Did that show independence?

I didn't know. I didn't own *The First Twelve Months*.

"You're better off without it," my friend Nancy said. "Supposedly, Harry should be sleeping through the night by now, and last night he got me up three times." She yawned. I did, too.

My daughter was no longer a newborn.

I took her to Zabar's in her Snugli. She was awake, alert, wide-eyed. But no one paid attention to her. No one doted on her; no one returned her innocent smile. Instead of looking at her as a precious new flower, people seemed to perceive her as one more snot-nosed kid. Perhaps, I thought, it was good for her to learn at an early age that she hadn't hung the moon.

Although, of course, she had.

My mother and I weren't spending much time together lately because Lewis was not feeling well and they were going back and forth to the hospital. He was undergoing frightening tests and was not up for company. They were afraid he might have lymphoma, and were talking about chemotherapy. She said that Lewis had begun to lose a lot of weight and, catching his reflection in the mirror, had cursed his "impatient skull." Not only did he not want to see people, but he didn't want to see people seeing him — didn't want to see them holding back tears, or crying, straining for small talk, or chatting too fast.

It was an ironic shame that just when my mother and I needed each other most, we saw each other least. I called and asked about Lewis; she called and asked about Elizabeth. She even baby-sat when I was really stuck. But there wasn't a lot of dropping by. I hoped Lewis would get well and at least decide to welcome visitors. And I hoped that in the meantime Mom would come find joy in my home with my child.

I hated this overlapping of sunrise and sunset. Hated that on some weird subconscious level, it might feel as though Elizabeth were pushing Lewis out of the picture, forcing my mother to grow old.

Here I'd been concerned that my mother would be too happy to be a doting grandmother. Instead, she was too miserable.

I felt disappointed, but guilty too. Lewis might have cancer. How dare I be let down that my mother wasn't a hands-and-knees grandmother. And how absurd. She had never been a hands-and-knees mom.

She had always been a working mother. When I was a young adult, I felt proud: Mom was my role model. When I was an adult, I felt lucky: Mom was my confidante. Now that I was a mother, what made me imagine that — presto — she'd fit into a more traditional mold? And why was I letting this bother me now, when Mom had disease and sorrow on her mind?

Mom revealed that while on weekdays she and Dad always kept us up late so they could play with us, after a weekend, she'd also feel Thank God It's Monday — she'd be ready to have some breathing room again. I laughed. It made sense. But I also felt a weird retroactive hurt.

This was crazy. I hadn't felt neglected thirty years ago. Why was I feeling it now? I had a mentor mother. How come I wanted a gushing grandma? One of those ladies who rushed over three afternoons a week to kidnap the baby?

I tried to be fair. I knew Mom's being a cab ride away had its drawbacks. It's easier to gush from afar. When you live ten minutes away, there's more pressure to follow through, and more possibility for disappointment. I knew, too, that I couldn't expect Mom to fuss and carry on as Dad would have, or worse, to stand in for both parents.

"I just wish you'd come visit more often," I said one day as she was stepping into the elevator.

"Well, honey, I don't want to meddle."

"Mom," my voice caught. "I *want* you to meddle!"

Suddenly I was in tears, her arms were around me, and the elevator was going down empty.

It's odd when you make your mother a grandmother. After childbirth, many women get along better than ever with their parents. Others have a period of uneasy transition.

My mother and I had always been close, and I felt selfish now for wanting more from her than she could give. She loved Elizabeth. Someday she'd probably be the kind of grandmother who would take Elizabeth on bird walks and to matinees. Why couldn't I be patient?

My mother wasn't baby crazy. She was a writer and an editor. She had encouraged me with words and sentences, if not toys and blocks. She had typed up my school papers and critiqued my first articles. I was grateful for that. But I was still confused about what I now expected from her and from myself.

What would I be for Elizabeth? Was it possible to be a role-model career woman and a cookie-baking mom? What would Elizabeth demand of me when it was my turn to grandmother her little one? Was it possible that all new mothers hope for more than is reasonable?

I was having an identity crisis. I was trying to buy a dress for my book tour, and I didn't know where to begin. I wanted to look hip enough so that teenage girls would listen to me but conservative enough so that their parents would trust me.

Everything I tried on made me feel schlumpy, frumpy, and dumpy. In Jaeger, I felt too young. In The Limited, I felt too old. Everywhere else on Madison Avenue, I felt too poor.

My baby-sitting time ran out and I came home depressed. Not only was I empty-handed, but my failure to find anything made me feel I wasn't sure who I was anymore. Or who I would be. I almost bought a skimpy summer dress, but then wondered if I might get pregnant again by fall.

I'd felt so good pregnant. Cute in my borrowed clothes. Fulfilled producing Elizabeth. Why didn't I feel equally fulfilled raising her? Why was I so down? Motherhood was bliss lined with drudgery, but I'd have to make peace with that, wouldn't I? Was I going through postpartum depression? Or predeparture blues? I didn't want to kiss my baby good-bye.

Weaning, even partial weaning, was both harder and easier than I'd imagined. Easier in that it didn't take long for my body to cut down to just three feedings a day. Harder in that it made me sad to offer a bottle when my breasts were full.

I'd soon be away on the tour, and though I planned to pump and didn't want to lose my milk completely, I also didn't want Elizabeth to go hungry.

I wasn't too worried. Though some babies say, "Breast or bust!" Elizabeth seemed happy with either milk or formula. In the words of the pediatrician: it made no difference.

The phone rang.

"Is this a bad time?" Ellen asked.

"Elizabeth is nursing and I'm editing, but hey . . ."

We talked. Elizabeth grunted. The word processor hummed.

I didn't know whether to feel good about simultaneously being friend, mother, and writer, or bad because I wasn't giving 100 percent to anything anymore.

A magazine accepted an essay I sent and assigned me to write a quiz, due in three weeks.

"Are you a full-time writer?" the editor asked.

"I always have been, but now I'm a full-time mother, too, and I'm trying to figure out how it all works. Do you have kids?"

"Yes. A two-year-old and a six-year-old." She said she also had a novel coming out in September.

"That's amazing! How do you manage?"

She laughed. "My slip shows all the time."

"So Gene is coming tomorrow?" I asked Rob.

"At one-thirty."

"Good thing Cubby is finally sleeping through the night," I said. "Rob, how do you think your mother was as a mother?"

He was silent as he offered Elizabeth her bottle. "Well, she always always always got shampoo in my eyes."

I studied him. "Other than that?"

"Other than that, she was perfect."

I wondered which of my shortcomings Elizabeth would never forgive me for. And which she'd inherit.

"Stay with her. I'm going to go deal with the mail." I went into my office to answer teen letters and fill in a questionnaire for my tenth-year college reunion. The fifth question read: "What is your greatest frustration? (1) Work (2) Personal relationship (3) Family life (4) Balancing work and family (5) Other."

That was easy. I checked "Balancing work and family," and went back to the living room. Rob was saying, "You have sweaty palms, Cupcake. That won't do at all when you're slow-dancing at the junior prom."

"How would you have answered this?" I interrupted and showed him the question.

"I don't know." He adjusted Elizabeth on his lap. "I don't have a greatest frustration. Work's fine and family's fine."

"And let me guess, the balance is fine." I couldn't help sounding cynical.

"That's why I hired you."

"Thin ice, buddy, thin ice."

I wondered how many other alumnae were answering as I was. Juggling was a female problem. Like PMS.

Yes, Rob did a lot of cooking and cleaning. But if he had a meeting, he knew I'd cover for him. If I had a meeting, I knew I had to scramble for child care. Same thing at night. If we had a party we were going to without Elizabeth, Rob didn't worry about hiring a sitter or making a deal with a neighbor. Rob worried about what to wear: his tweed jacket or his wool one.

My bags were packed for the book tour and I hugged my four-month-old good-bye. My eyes misted over and I prayed all the planes would stay up. "If I die, show her the videos and scrapbooks so she knows I loved her."

"Don't even say that."

I wasn't trying to be morbid. I didn't want to die before Elizabeth grew up. But I couldn't help imagining the worst. I reminded Rob that we had to redo our will and choose a guardian.

"And Gene, thanks again for coming." She'd arrived the day before and had handed me innumerable glasses of water, saying she remembered how thirsty she got while nursing. "Take good care of Elizabeth."

I was off. Off to Pittsburgh, Cleveland, Columbus, Indianapolis, Minneapolis, Houston, and Dallas. I had bought a royal blue dress and had figured out what I wanted to say about AIDS, drugs, broken hearts, and first dates. I was ready for the firing line.

But I wasn't ready to leave Elizabeth. During the trip, I showed my brag book of her photos to airplane passengers, media escorts, bellhops, waiters, producers, reporters, interns, and other touring authors. I also looked at the photos alone in my hotel rooms.

You'd think I would have enjoyed the time away, the chance to read, drink wine, eat junk food, sleep uninterrupted. And I did. But it was almost too early for a great escape. Despite my conflicting feelings about motherhood, I was now mother first, writer second. The books I'd taken along weren't detective novels but parenting guides. And when talk show hosts asked me about teens, I sometimes wanted to tell them about babies.

What did I know about teens anyway? "The parents of a boy

worry about their boy," I told a newspaper reporter. "The parents of a girl worry about every boy in town."

"Heap on the praise. Choose your quarrels well," I told a women's group. "Arm your teens with information: what they don't know *can* hurt them. Tell them you feel awkward talking about it, tell them you hope they'll wait, but tell them about contraception. One million teens get pregnant each year."

My message and delivery were fine. But was I on automatic pilot? I wondered how I'd feel when Elizabeth was older. Would I know more about raising teens when she was a teen? Or would I know more about her, but less about adolescents at large? Would I be as adamant about discussing birth control? Maybe the distance now served me well.

Between cities, I used the breast pump in airport lavatories and flushed the milk down toilets. I hated feeling like Elsie the Cow doing a trombone solo. That was the worst part of the tour.

The best part wasn't playing know-it-all, getting made up to go on T.V., chancing upon a celebrity in the green room, or having a short-lived expense account. It was being able to visit far-flung cousins and friends. When the tour was over, I spent an extra day in Texas to be with my grandfather.

There I stopped again at my father's grave. It had been almost a year since the last visit. I cried, as I have each time I've gone to the cemetery. And I showed him Elizabeth's photographs. I knew it was inane to flash her pictures at the ground. I figured Dad either knew about Elizabeth (a comforting thought I wished I could believe) or he didn't. Either way, I vowed again, she would know about him.

On the airplane home I sat next to a woman who said she was thirty-three and had been married six years. I showed her my well-worn brag book.

"I know what I should want and I know what I want to

want, but I'm not ready. I imagine I'll wake up one day and suddenly want to get pregnant," she said. "Or maybe my mother will call me and say, 'It's time.' Right now, I like my freedom and my life-style and I like being able to afford pretty much anything I want."

I told her my husband had to talk me into it but that I was glad he did. "You know in *The Wizard of Oz* how it suddenly goes from black-and-white to color? Well, the change isn't that dramatic. It's not like your life is one-dimensional until kids come along. But I love love love my daughter — and objectively, she's not even interesting yet. Being a mother takes a lot of energy and expense, but I wouldn't miss it for anything."

I told her I was forming this strange new view of rich and poor, of haves and have-nots. "I know this lady, Inez, who has seven kids, and it practically makes me wistful. I'll probably stop at two or three, but I've caught myself envying mothers with big families."

She looked at me like I was crazy. "I think I'm afraid of childbirth," she confessed.

"Who isn't? We all saw *Gone with the Wind*. But that's why there are drugs. Then the pain is gone, and you get to keep the baby."

"Don't they cry all the time at first?"

"No. A few definitely do. But babies have a bad rap. Even changing diapers is no big deal, and that just lasts a few years." I was beginning to believe that maybe time flies whether you're having fun or not, so you might as well have fun *and* have babies. Besides, if you don't have them when you are young, you won't have them when you are old.

"How long did it take you to lose the weight you'd gained?"

"I still can't zip up all my pants. But I'm getting there." She was missing the point. "Look, I have a baby. Who needs a waistline?" I handed my tray to the flight attendant. "It's none of my business, but if you want a family, I wouldn't wait forever because your fertility and your energy level are just going to go down."

God I was a pain in the ass. I wondered if it was 95 percent because I believed what I said — and 5 percent because misery loves company.

I got home after midnight. Elizabeth was asleep, but I nudged her awake and put her to my breast. She nursed contentedly. I was relieved to know that I hadn't gone dry, that our dance was not over, that I hadn't sacrificed this closeness for the sake of my career.

Not that she smiled or offered any sign of recognition.

Having grown used to rapid-fire interviews and televised tête-à-têtes, I had expected some reaction, some grunt of gratitude, despite the hour. But Elizabeth was still a baby. And four-month-olds, I had to remind myself, are more indifferent than intense. Besides, if she was too young to notice I was back, maybe she was too young to notice I'd been gone.

My cat never threw a welcome-home party for me either, but I knew she liked having me around.

I climbed into bed.

"Hi, Rob," I whispered.

"Hi. How'd it go?"

"Fine. I'll tell you tomorrow. How were things here?"

"Gene left yesterday and today I felt like Mr. Mom." He gave me a kiss. "Cub care is hard work."

Now he'd know why I got so desperate at the end of each day. "Did Gene have fun?"

"With her son and granddaughter? She was in pig heaven."

"I just nursed Elizabeth. I don't think she even missed me, but I missed her."

The tour was over, rain ticked against the window, Chanda purred at my shoulder, Elizabeth slept in the next room, and I began making love with my husband, the father of my child. "This is my family," I thought. "This is where I am in my life."

I couldn't get enough of Elizabeth. My time away from her helped me enjoy my time with her. Rob had had his fill of shining eyes and kicking feet and was eager to take off. But I

wanted nothing more than to hang out with my baby, to admire her, read to her, make faces at her. To take her to the park
and let her work the crowd. To bathe her and let her splash. I
put her down and watched her pull out her pacifier, then fuss
when she couldn't put it back in. When she slept I actually
missed her — though I remembered well that I usually found
her nap as precious as her smile.

That night Rob lifted Elizabeth and crowed "Woo! Woo!
Woo!" She twinkled, smiled, then actually giggled — a first.
Rob and I looked at each other with tears in our eyes. Our
daughter was learning to laugh. To laugh! We had made a little
person who was able to experience joy. And able to create it.

I took notes at an all-day meeting of the American Society of Journalists and Authors. My career was a caricature. I'd started writing for *Seventeen*, moved on to *Glamour* and *Cosmo*, paused at *Bride's* and *Modern Bride*, headed toward *Redbook*, *Woman's Day*, *Ladies' Home Journal*, and *McCall's*, and was now working on articles for *Parenting* and *American Baby*. My brothers kidded me that *Modern Maturity* was next and that my last essay would be "Going Out in Style" for *The Mortician's Gazette*.

Yet at the end of the conference, I knew I wasn't going to fire off any new proposals. I was going to tickle Elizabeth's toes and try to get her to laugh again.

For a brief moment, for better and worse, my ambition had lost its edge. I needed a mix of writing and mothering, but I didn't know how many parts of one to stir with how many of the other. And I didn't know that the formula would keep changing according to my baby's age and my interests and energy.

I did know that life is long and kids grow up. That there would be time to tell stories, but that babies don't stay babies. I wanted to ride high on Elizabeth's and my rekindled love affair, on the smiling and the staring.

For now it felt right to revel in the life of the home. I often wished that I didn't often wish for more.

My friend Nancy quit work to spend time with her two boys. We were going down her elevator. "I was ordering some toy from a catalog," she said, "and the lady asked me for my home phone and my work number. I almost went into a dog-and-pony show about how I used to work, and how I would work again, but I was just taking a little time off. I was all defensive. It was nuts!"

I laughed. I understood.

I was trying to stay relaxed. Trying not to pick up speed. Trying not to worry about my career clock or the loss of professional momentum. Yet I kept all too busy when Elizabeth was awake *and* when she was asleep. Days still had only twenty-four hours, and I was attempting to squeeze my old life and my new life into the same short period.

I hired Matilde to spend ten hours a week with Elizabeth instead of just six. But I still didn't know how to find room for Elizabeth and work, Rob and rest. And me.

Part of the problem was that writing and mothering don't start and stop. You can never leave either behind. You can always do both a little more, a little better.

You can also drive yourself crazy.

I knew I had a lot to learn from the park-bench moms.

Elizabeth and I went to Riverside Park at nine o'clock one morning. I sat on a bench; she sat on me. Together we watched the park come to life. Squirrels darted from tree to tree. Dog walkers made their loops. A French nanny said hello. So did a Chinese student.

We watched a play group. Four-year-olds formed a ring and mimicked their instructor. They touched their toes and said, "I am an elevator and I'm stopping at the basement." They put their hands on their knees and said, "I am an elevator and I'm stopping at the first floor." They touched their second-floor waists and third-floor shoulders and fourth-floor heads. Finally, before disbanding, they stretched their hands high and cried in unison, "I am an elevator and I'm stopping at the penthouse."

Elizabeth studied this urban folklore and gummed her favorite duck toy.

When we left the park, a ragged fellow asked me her name, reached into his pocket, and gave her a quarter.

"Oh, you don't have to do that," I said.

He hunched his shoulders. "I want to."

I thanked him and felt the weight of the coin. I couldn't just add it to the nickels and dimes in my pocket, so I decided to use it to begin Elizabeth's first piggy bank.

Back home, we got into our own elevator. It was brand new; it beeped on every floor, for the benefit of the blind. Elizabeth and the other babies in the building loved the beeping. She also loved when other passengers entered the car. She'd flap her arms, squeal with mirth, and behave as though long-lost friends were dropping by for tea.

I was beginning to wonder if elevators are to city kids what backyards are to suburban ones.

There's nothing like a baby in its bathwater. Some parents get sore backs washing their kids. Not me. I hopped right in with Elizabeth. I enjoyed taking my bath with her and she enjoyed it, too. It was a time when I focused on her entirely instead of also trying to read or talk on the phone or answer mail. We'd play with her toys and sing special bath-time songs.

Once I heard myself singing "Oh, I wish I were a little bar of soap," a line I hadn't thought of in decades. It was from a ditty that my mother sang to me, and her mother sang to her, and her mother probably sang to her, silly joyful words now echoing through the years.

I also bounced Elizabeth between my knees and, more or less to the tune of the *Beverly Hillbillies* theme, sang a song I'd made up:

I'm Captain Elizabeth, I'm going for a ride;
I'm Captain Elizabeth, I'm going side to side;
I'm Captain Elizabeth, I'm going up and down;
I'm Captain Elizabeth, I'm going round and round;
I'm Captain Elizabeth, I'm going back and forth;
I'm Captain Elizabeth, I'm going south and north;
I'm Captain Elizabeth, I'm head of my whole crew;
I'm Captain Elizabeth, and I love you.

It wasn't much, but she loved it, and it soon became a ritual.

Bedtime had rituals of its own. I'd tell her about her day, sing "Good Night Elizabeth," to the tune of "Good Night Ladies," give her a pacifier, kiss her, and dim her light, ever grateful to Rob for having installed the dimmer.

There were nights when Elizabeth cried. It was hard to walk out on her then. Even when I knew that she was beyond tired. Even when I knew that, if left alone, her tears would last only a few minutes. Even when I knew that the kindest thing would be to let her cry, let her find her way to sleep.

Getting her to sleep always seemed to be my elusive goal. And that sometimes made me feel guilty.

I called Susan, whose baby was due any minute. "I love Elizabeth, but I always want her to go to sleep," I confessed. "Is something wrong with me? Is that like a death wish?"

"Don't be ridiculous. It's a sleep wish."

I came across this passage in Don DeLillo's *White Noise:*

> Watching children sleep makes me feel devout, part of a spiritual system. It is the closest I can come to God. If there is a secular equivalent of standing in a great spired cathedral with marble pillars and streams of mystical light slanting through two-tier Gothic windows, it would be watching children in their little bedrooms fast asleep. Girls especially.

I knew what he meant. Rob and I both liked to check on Elizabeth all evening long. Sometimes one of us would suggest, "Let's wake her up and play with her." But we knew we were kidding. Watching her sleep provided the joy without the work. We could rejoice that we had her without having to actually deal with her.

Sometimes we'd go into her room to hang a blanket over her window in the hope that the darkness would buy an extra hour in the morning. Sometimes we'd go in to put away clothes or to look for something in her chest of drawers. I always turned on the hall light, tiptoed in with the door ajar, then waited for my eyes to adjust to the silver sliver filtering in. Rob's method was to charge inside and flick on the overhead track lights, dimmer be damned. "She can sleep through anything," he'd assure me, planting a peck on her cheek.

He was usually right. But when he was wrong, I'd remind him of the house rules: You woke her, you bought her.

Our friend Arlene had a baby boy: Christopher. The birth took about two hours, tops.

Susan also had a baby boy: Rafael. The birth was hard. Endless hours of labor followed by a C-section. A double whammy. But Susan was deliriously happy and enjoyed a postpartum elation that lasted for months.

We were honored to be asked to Rafael's *bris*, though we felt a little funny about witnessing the event. Not because of Susan and Miguel's interfaith marriage (she's Jewish, he's Catholic), but because we'd never been privy to the snipping of a foreskin. The *mohel* spoke English and Hebrew, pronounced the Spanish name fairly well, then did the deed. Pomp and circumcision. Rafael scarcely cried. The adults, however, looked plenty nervous. Especially the men.

Rob and I watched an episode of *thirtysomething* in which Hope and Michael left baby Janey behind and went on a getaway to reignite their passion.

It sparked an argument between us. Spring was here, skirts were short, Rob was randy. We had sex two nights in a row (I was perpetually tired and thought I deserved a medal), and on night three, Rob was ready to go. I said no and he launched into a "the passion is gone" number and threw in that we didn't go out much anymore.

"Whoa," I protested. "Michael took Hope on a quickie second honeymoon and ordered room service champagne. He didn't just turn off the T.V. and pounce. Besides, you have a short memory. And we do, too, go out."

I was more comfortable with life's phases than Rob. I didn't mind coasting along pleasantly, sinking softly into the armchair of Time. I didn't expect sex to be at the same feverish pitch it was years earlier. And I'd lost my taste for loud bars and clubs.

Wasn't the main point of going out finding someone with whom to stay in?

According to the *Village Voice*, Dr. Ruth was doing a show on sex before and after pregnancy. I rounded up my new-mother friends and announced that we were going on a field trip.

We filed into the front row of the studio and started whispering about sex before the show even began. Ashley, like me, wished her desire would come back. Leslie said she gave her son so many kisses and hugs all day that she was rarely in the mood when it was her husband's turn. And then there was Susan, the newest mother among us, but also, apparently, the most libidinous. Neither tired nor headachy, she'd been feeling extra loving lately. She and Miguel had even gotten personal while she was still in the hospital, thank you very much.

Lights, camera, action. Dr. Ruth strutted on stage and interviewed an ob/gyn and a pregnant actress. Then she faced us, her audience, and next thing you know, I was telling all on national T.V. "When we were trying to conceive, my husband and I had good sex because it seemed important and purposeful," I began. "When we were expecting, we often had good sex because we didn't use birth control and because my husband liked my changing figure," I continued. "But now that we have our baby, I spend all day cuddling her and I just don't have the appetite my husband does. When my ob/gyn said we'd have to wait six weeks before resuming relations, I wished he'd told us to wait longer." My heart was pounding. "So this is what I want to know: when will my lust come back?"

"Vonderful question!" Dr. Ruth chimed and turned to her expert of the hour. It was odd being an anonymous audience member when I had so recently been in the interviewee's hot seat.

"Breast-feeding affects hormones," the ob/gyn explained. "Couples use so much K-Y jelly at this time that they go sliding around the bedroom."

The audience laughed.

A fine sound bite, but I hadn't asked about lubrication. I'd asked about lust.

A gigantic pregnant woman to my right squealed, "Six weeks! I won't be able to wait six weeks."

"You may be surprised," Ashley and Leslie piped in. Susie-Q-sie just smiled.

The woman then revealed that she "breast-fed" her husband. "I have a lot of milk," she said to the camera. "Can I continue breast-feeding my husband even after the baby arrives?"

"Sure," said the ob/gyn, "but feed the baby first."

The audience roared.

It was a fun outing, but also unsettling. The show was a celebration of wonderful sex. But it was a little too pat. Instead of reassuring pregnant women and new moms that it was okay not to feel horny round the clock, it extolled the wonders of K-Y jelly and reminded women that they could gratify their men without engaging in intercourse. Nothing wrong with that, but I wish someone had pointed out that there is also nothing wrong with saying a guiltless no from time to time.

And I wish the ob/gyn had told me what I would soon learn: this, too, would pass. Lust does return — but sometimes not until after the baby is weaned, after the mother is rested, after her body is her own again.

Elizabeth was five months old. She could shriek. She could prop herself up and turn from her belly to her back. She liked tummy kisses, playing with blocks, peekaboo, and the Eensie Weensie Spider. She liked her duck doll Squeaky and her new walker-stroller. She liked her playpen. (Mothers told me if I didn't use the playpen early, she'd consider it a cage.) She often laughed and sometimes fussed. (Fussed. Now *there* was a euphemism.) And she was starting to outgrow outfits she'd hardly worn.

The pediatrician weighed her in at almost fourteen pounds and said to try her on rice and cereals.

"Where do I get them?"

"You know the aisle in the grocery store that you never go down?" he asked. "There."

He said I could also start her on solid foods, "mashed bananas or jarred fruits or yellow vegetables."

"How much should I feed her?"

"I can't tell you what size steak to eat," he said. "As long as she keeps opening her mouth — within reason — you can keep shoveling it in." He also said to offer one food at a time, allowing three days before introducing each so that I could tell if she had any adverse reaction.

I did. She didn't.

Her first square meal was one spoonful of oatmeal mixed with three of warm formula. Mmmm. Though much of it landed on her bib, she seemed to think food was a pretty swell idea. But it took several weeks before she acquired a real taste for strained peaches, pears, or sweet potatoes. And several more before ripe avocado spooned straight from the fruit became her staple of choice.

"You never told me how hard it is," Arlene said on the phone. Christopher peeped in the background.

216

"You never told me how great it is," Susan said on the phone. Rafael peeped in the background.

"Oh yes I did," I answered them both. I'd told them motherhood was difficult and wonderful and fulfilling and frustrating. I'd told them it was like having an adorable puppy you had to play with all the time. I'd told them that being a mother meant that if my baby slept poorly, I slept poorly. That if Rob worked extra-long hours, I worked extra-long hours. That if Rob said he wanted to sign up for volleyball, my first thought was, "On whose clock?" I'd told them that he and I had always been nice to each other, but that now we kept score. I'd even told them that I sometimes looked at my sleeping daughter — the curve of her nose, the arc of her ear — and found her so astonishingly beautiful that I hoped someday a husband would share her pillow and look at her with such awe, such unconditional love.

I'd told them motherhood was thrilling and tedious and time-consuming. I'd told them it was a mix of sunshine and shadow.

My friend Claudia interviewed me for a magazine article she was writing about how friendships change after a woman has a baby. Do new mothers inadvertently bore old pals? Is it painful for couples who want kids to be around couples who have them? Do new mothers really make new friends?

"Yes," I said, starting at the end. One way to meet men, single women are told, is to walk a dog. One way to meet mothers, I found, was to carry a baby. People were so friendly in the park that I sometimes had to remind myself that just because another woman and I were pushing swings side by side didn't mean we had to become soul mates.

Of course, I was grateful for Ashley, Leslie, Carol Ann, Karen, Bernadette, and the other moms in our building. They were good company and a good source for toys and tips. Some had their children on tight schedules; others were winging it.

We were all quietly showing each other that parenting had no absolutes.

Old friends? We had more in common than ever with the ones who were also parents. I liked being able to compare notes on food and diapers and not having to apologize if Elizabeth howled during dinner.

Most of my childless friends still seemed to call and care, too. I tried not to bore them with the minutiae of Elizabeth's day (she slept four hours and pooped four times and drank four ounces of formula . . .). And I tried not to be feeding her or playing with her when I was on the phone. But nor did I want to have long chats during my child-care time or Elizabeth's nap time.

When old friends talked about goings-on in the office and out, I sometimes felt I had to stretch for something interesting to say. When they asked if I was doing any writing, I'd mention my journal or some magazine assignment, but would wind up feeling defensive. (You try writing on choppy sleep and ten hours a week of child care!) When they didn't ask — didn't acknowledge my professional side — I also felt defensive. (I still have aspirations; I still care about words.)

It wasn't easy. But for the most part we were weathering this period of change. I particularly warmed to friends who warmed to Elizabeth and appreciated those who were accommodating, who were willing to come over for a simple dinner instead of hoping I'd meet them at a restaurant.

Patty and I started walking instead of jogging. Sometimes she even pushed the stroller.

Seth was busy in med school but still made time for a quick stopover or an occasional picnic lunch in the park.

And I was always comfortable with Meredith. She knew about kids because of her nephews, and she was great both at roughhousing and quiet play.

What about Beth and Ed? That friendship could have come unglued if we'd let it. But we all liked each other and they had our baby charmed. Ed often had a harmonica in his pocket, which Elizabeth eventually learned to ask for. Every few times we went out — but not every time — we asked them how *it* was going. They still hadn't conceived, and talking about it made more sense than ignoring the Elephant in the Living Room. They knew we were rooting for them. And they weren't despairing. They loved each other and their jobs and their friends and their friends' kids, and as Ed pointed out, "We're having fun trying."

The only person I was losing was Valerie. Neither of us wanted to weed the other from our garden of friends. But when I spoke to her — briefly — about weaning, she said, "I can't relate." And I couldn't relate to her life in the fast lane. I no longer wanted to meet for dinner at nine or a party at ten. That was too close to bedtime.

Maybe someday we'd drift back together. Or maybe when family takes the lead, a friendship or two always falls behind.

At five and a half months, Elizabeth went to her first baseball game. On the subway to Yankee Stadium, Rob carried her in a Snugli and a man offered him his seat. Rob accepted, flustered but gracious.

We bought reserved tickets for ourselves and two friends from Barcelona, but we couldn't get four seats together. When we reached the stands, we decided to ignore our ticket numbers and spotted four seats in a row. We were about to settle in with our hot dogs, popcorn, potato chips, and beer.

An usher challenged us. "I can't let you sit here."

"We paid the full amount," Rob said, "and we'll leave if the people come."

"I can't let you sit here."

"This is my first game," our friend Teresa said. "We came all the way from Spain."

"I can't let you sit here. My supervisor is watching."

"It's her first game, too." Rob pointed to Elizabeth. She smiled on cue.

"Don't do this to me," the usher said. "I'm a softie."

"Please," we all pleaded in unison.

He shot a glance to where his supervisor had been standing. "Okay, sit down. Hurry."

We thanked him and cheered the Yankees on to victory. Elizabeth didn't cry or nap. She loved the seventh-inning stretch. She flirted shamelessly with other fans (she's always been partial to men). She gleefully crinkled her unopened bag of chips. And she and I played at conversation: I blew against her arm and she blew against mine.

I'd never enjoyed a baseball game so much. Being part of a family was even more fun than being part of a couple.

Elizabeth also attended her first free concert in Central Park. We picnicked as we listened to the Metropolitan Opera perform

L'Elisir d'amore and watched escaped balloons fly past the clouds and moon. It was a perfect summer evening. Not only was Luciano Pavarotti there, but so was Ed Koch, who was mayor at the time.

When I spotted him stepping his way around blankets and folding chairs, I grabbed Elizabeth and jogged toward him.

"You're a politician. This is a baby. You know what to do."

He did. He kissed her without missing a beat.

Was Elizabeth quiet during the opera? For the most part. But then she suddenly had enough of bottles and pacifiers, and decided to accompany Pavarotti.

We decided to make a run for it.

On our answering machine was this message:

"This is for Elizabeth. If you want what you ordered, remember it's a cash-only transaction. Meet me on the corner of Eighty-eighth and Broadway at three o'clock. The stuff has never been cut, and I guarantee one hundred percent purity."

I laughed as I recognized the voice of my friend Masello. If Elizabeth ever really got a message like that, I'd have her head.

At almost six months, she still looked like both of us — little diplomat. She was getting better at sitting, rolling, reaching. She was beginning to hang on to Teddy, the bear Gene had given her when she was born. In general, she ignored her fancy toys and focused instead on buttons on her clothing and ribbons on her blanket.

Rob and I continued to be impressed by her every gesture. We also tried not to spook each other by wondering aloud, "What if she never develops beyond this?"

The day before her half-birthday, Elizabeth was not her jolly self. She'd gotten up on the wrong side of the crib and was grumpy, distraught, and weepy. At lunch, she was finishing a bottle and falling asleep. I was looking forward to eating and reading during her nap, but thought I'd get one little burp out of her first. I tapped her back. Tap tap tap. Tap tap tap.

She burped. Perfect.

Then she followed through with a power boot, spewing a full bottle of formula all over my shirt, my pants, my feet, her shirt, her legs, the sofa, the rug. My stomach was still empty, and now hers was, too. Plus I had laundry to do. Never a dull moment.

Teething. My poor child was drooling, putting her fingers in her mouth and chewing desperately on the frozen teething rings I began handing her. I offered Orajel, but nothing seemed to work.

At about 10:00 P.M., at the end of this, her Longest Day, up pointed two tiny tooth tops.

Cutest little saw-edged things you ever did see.

The next day Elizabeth was a happy camper again. Ashley and Matilde couldn't wait to peek inside her mouth.

"Let me see," Ashley said in English.

"*A ver*," Matilde said in Spanish.

I tried prying her mouth open. But the best way to get Elizabeth to show off her pearly whites was to make her smile or laugh — one of my favorite hobbies anyway. I tickled her, and she bared her baby teeth to great fanfare and applause.

I really liked Matilde. So did Elizabeth. She kicked and made high-pitched noises whenever I knocked on Ashley's door. Not only were the child-care hours good for my career and my sanity, but also, I felt, for Elizabeth's development. I liked it that while I was writing, Elizabeth was playing. And hearing Spanish. I liked it that Matilde's sunshine was helping her learn to trust and love other people.

But I never knew what to call Matilde. She was more than a baby-sitter, but not quite a nanny and not an au pair. Caregiver sounded pretentious. Friend was coy. Matilde, I finally decided, was Elizabeth's Significant Other.

Sometimes I'd drop in unexpectedly and Eliakim would be having lunch while Elizabeth would just be parked in the swing, pacifier in mouth. (I didn't entertain her every minute either.) Other times, I'd hear her laughing as I approached Ashley's door.

That day I heard music playing. I knocked loudly, and Matilde let me in. Eliakim was asleep in her crib, and Matilde was carrying Elizabeth, who was flapping and squealing and smiling radiantly.

"We were dancing," Matilde said, a little embarrassed.

"That's great! I don't dance with her enough."

Boxes of picture books had been arriving for the *Redbook*

contest, and Elizabeth and I had been doing lots of reading. But while I was all for book learning, I was mighty glad someone was asking my daughter to dance, too.

Elizabeth tried her new teeth out on me. "No!" I said — a word I probably didn't use often enough. "Do not bite the breast that feeds you," I explained, but she'd already burst into tears and now refused to continue.

Our nursing days were numbered. Fact was, she loved her bottle, whereas she could take or leave me. When I offered my breast, she often balked. When she didn't, when she acquiesced, it felt like a gift, a farewell embrace. Even then, she sometimes suckled against me and then, still unsatisfied, cried for more. I was becoming little more than a snack.

For whom was I doing this, anyway?

Elizabeth was ready to declare her independence. I'd have to accept that, ready or not.

It would be a difficult lesson, and one I'd surely have to learn again and again. Mothering, at any stage, is hard work. If you do your job well, your child needs you less. If you do your job right, your child gains confidence and wings.

I was about to have my body back. Would I welcome it? I could soon start drinking again. Did I want to? My blouses would no longer be misbuttoned, and I could wear dresses instead of just separates. Did I care?

My daughter could not yet walk or talk, and already I was growing nostalgic.

Why?

Because letting go begins with weaning.

Because letting go never really ends.

Part Four

Fast Forward

This book has been mostly about beginnings, but there were endings, too.

Lewis died midsummer. Cancer. To me, it seemed he went fast. To my mother, it must not have seemed that way. She was with him every moment, every day after day of his dying. Whereas my father's death had caught her by surprise, this time she had the chance to say good-bye and say it well.

Not that it helped much. Mom, widowed again, said she felt "like a piñata that's been beaten empty": all the fun was gone. She took some comfort in knowing that, at the end, Lewis had "wanted out," that he had "transcended" the respirator doctors had put him on. But she was flattened. She quoted a line he'd written in a play he'd been working on: "I've come to realize the only close death you ever get over is your own."

The memorial service was crowded with friends, including many long-married couples who had offered their condolences years ago when Dad died. One speaker, writer William Honan, said, "Lewis Bergman was truly a great editor because he cast out fresh and scintillating ideas the way a shaggy dog, emerging from a swim, shakes itself and makes the air glisten and sparkle." Rob read a poem, "The Long Boat," written by Stanley Kunitz, Lewis's Provincetown neighbor. It begins, "When his boat snapped loose from its moorings . . ." and ends:

> endlessly drifting.
> Peace! Peace!
> To be rocked by the Infinite!
> As if it didn't matter
> which way was home;
> as if he didn't know
> he loved the earth so much
> he wanted to stay forever.

My mother was preparing to make a final pilgrimage to Cape Cod, where she would say more good-byes, and help Lewis's grown son and daughter sell their house. But first she had to run a grim errand: she had to pick up Lewis's ashes. She wanted to take them north, to offer them to the rosebushes of his summer place and the waters of the Atlantic.

I met her at the funeral home. The box marked Bergman was incongruously small. In the taxi back to my mother's apartment, she held Lewis in her lap while I held Elizabeth in mine. "We're going home," she told him.

Chanda died several weeks later. I was in Armonk with Mom, Rob, Elizabeth, and my brother Mark, in the house where we grew up. A neighbor in our building was looking in on Chanda. Poor cat had developed a kidney infection and had virtually stopped eating. The neighbor phoned and said, "You better come in. She's not looking well." But by the time we got everybody piled into the car and back in the city, it was too late. Chanda was stretched on the sofa, languorous, but stiff, and with her eyes open.

I was sad, and sorry I wasn't with her at the end. I knew some animals preferred to die alone, but I felt I'd let her down. I was glad she died at home, though, and I wasn't as broken up as I would have been had she died even a year earlier. Elizabeth's birth and Lewis's death put Chanda's life into perspective. She lived to be eighteen and a half. It was time for her.

We placed Chanda in a box and Mom told me to put in a note. She knew about my good-byes, and she knew Chanda had seen me through most of my life, from first kiss to first death to first baby.

"I'll take her home and bury her out back in Armonk," Mom volunteered. That's where our less long-lived cats were buried: Pokey, Smokey, the Pussy Pumpkins I and II. I thanked her. I didn't want to call the pet crematorium.

"Dig really deep, and put on lots of stones," I said, sniffling. "Remember how dogs tried to dig up Smokey?"

The burial would be hard for Mom. It would feel like the end of an era. Mom had been through so much. And Chanda was her cat, too. Like me, Mom remembered when Dad brought her home — long ago, when our family was young.

For us, day followed night, and life went on. By the time Elizabeth had spent nine months inside me and nine months out, her dark baby hair was long gone, replaced by short fine wisps of chestnut brown. She had big ears and pinchable Dizzy Gillespie cheeks, and her arched eyebrows set off blue eyes, which were sometimes round with innocence, sometimes bright with mischief and fun.

Elizabeth had learned, if not mastered, a great many things. She could say "mama" and "book." She could say "bye-bye" and wave. She could hold her bottle. She could clap her hands. She could pull herself up and knock things down. She could demonstrate her injured-grasshopper crawl. She could yank off her father's glasses and her mother's clip-on earrings. She could even entertain indulgent friends by engaging in heavy breathing on the phone.

She had also begun to grind her teeth (all four of them). She had discovered her nostrils (to her delight and my chagrin). She had survived her first fall (a thud from the living-room sofa when both Rob and I were home — there is nothing more dangerous than the diffusion of responsibility).

She had already visited her great-grandfather in Texas. And she had been christened in her great-grandmother's baby dress — made by a great-great-grandmother — in Manhattan's French church, *L'Eglise Française du Saint Esprit*. Meredith was her godmother, and Seth, who had just married Lucie, was her godfather.

Elizabeth had occasional tantrums, times when we complained that she was "being a baby" or having a "Lizzie Tizzie." But like most babies, she was usually good-natured. She loved bubble-blowing, board books, Raffi songs, burrowing in wastebaskets, unpacking boxes and drawers, playing patty-cake and Pease Porridge Hot, wiggling to country music, swinging in the park, and practicing the *m*-word.

When she was babbling and Rob was nearby, I'd ask, "Who's your favorite parent?" and she'd say, "Mamamamamama." He was only half amused. He could still make her laugh more readily than I, but she clung to me — sometimes even when Rob wanted to play and I wanted a break.

Elizabeth also began weekly sessions at Gymboree exercise class. I had attended an open house only because it was free and nearby. Alas, her eyes lit up when the instructor sang "Parachute Time," "Tick Tock Tick Tock," and "The More We Get Together, the Happier We'll Be." Who was I to deprive my kid of midday bubbles, tunnels, seesaws, and slides? I signed up and plunked down a hefty chunk of change.

Gymboree was designed not just for babies to meet babies, but for moms to meet moms. My new neighbor friends and I were beginning to talk about setting up a basement playroom and a weekly story hour. Yet some of the mothers were already fleeing the city. Ashley was moving to Pennsylvania. Leslie was off to New Jersey. Nancy was headed for the suburbs. I figured it wouldn't hurt to make new friends.

One Gymboree mother asked how much I fed Elizabeth.

"Oh, it varies day to day." I mentioned some of her favorite foods (avocado, tortellini, Cheerios) and added that I'd been careful to stay away from the ones doctors said to avoid: honey, eggs, grapes, nuts, hot dogs.

She proceeded to delineate her precise system of getting necessary nutrients down her child. "I run a tight ship," she concluded, making me feel that mine had holes.

Meeting other moms, I began to realize, could be overrated.

I met nannies, too. Some looked bored, but most seemed to enjoy watching their charges bounce on the trampoline or pound on the xylophone. I overheard one say to another, "I'd never be a working mother. We get all the good stuff."

At almost ten months, Elizabeth started saying "dada." When Rob put on his jacket each morning, she'd look at him with blueberry eyes, say "bye-bye," then dissolve into tears as he went down the elevator. I wasn't sure if she was sad that he was leaving for work or worried that he'd vaporize once the doors shut.

Sometimes she and I would head off to a museum. Never have I been so culturally caught up, and I came to consider museum-hopping one of the privileges of motherhood. I also tried to plan lunch dates, errands with friends, or jaunts to the zoo to break up the routine and fend off boredom.

Of course lunch out had its perils. One day I met Ed near his office. We searched for a restaurant with a high chair or sassy seat ("No, that's a booster seat; she's not old enough for a booster seat"), and finally found an accommodating diner. As I took a stab at adult conversation, Elizabeth made mealtime a hands-on experience. She had a party smearing herself with yogurt and applesauce, then proceeded to drop toys, forks, spoons, and sugar packets on the ground in an enthralling game of Mommy Pick-Up. She'd let go of each item and watch it fall; I'd bend down and retrieve it.

"The girl's gifted," Ed said. "A regular little Isaac Newton. If she'd just come up with this a few hundred years ago, it could have been Elizabeth's law of gravity."

Where had I read that Goethe said, "If children grew up according to early indications, we should have nothing but geniuses"? I gave Elizabeth a Sweet 'n' Low and a kiss. "She's gifted at making messes," I said.

Back home I learned once again that the best way to tell if a kid's diaper is dirty is by taking a peek, not a poke. The phone rang just as I'd gotten Elizabeth onto the changing table. I hurriedly changed her, then ran around trying to find the cordless phone. (Where had I put it?) By the time I located it, the answering-machine message had begun. "Hold on," I shouted. Elizabeth pressed redial, and the caller had to wait for seven more notes to sound. "Hello," I finally said.

It was Rob. I recognized his laugh. "We're not real professional around here," I said, "but we get to every call."

I told Rob about lunch and said that Elizabeth had given me her first kiss. "You know how I always say, 'Mommy loves Elizabeth, Mommy hugs Elizabeth, Mommy kisses Elizabeth?' Well, today she leaned her little wet mouth against my cheek."

Rob was glad he'd caught me in a good mood because he was calling to say he'd be working late. Again.

I had a terrific husband. He was never around. I had a terrific kid. She was always around.

It was only three-thirty and already I was out of steam. "Why don't you watch *Sesame Street?*" I suggested to Elizabeth and put her in front of the T.V. "I'm going to work — or conk out — and I'll be back in an hour." Elizabeth looked at the tube and looked at me as if to say, "Dream on, Mom."

I called Patty and she agreed to meet me for a walk in the park. We were a few minutes late because Elizabeth went rigid and sway back as I tried to buckle her in her stroller. Worse, I think she sensed that her early assertiveness amused me as much as it annoyed me.

"I'm tired," I told Patty, explaining that Elizabeth slept twelve hours at night but only one during the day. "It's not easy. I'd hoped I'd be wise enough to remember that I had my whole life to be a writer and that Elizabeth's infancy is precious and fleeting."

"Eleven hours isn't fleeting," Patty said. How come I kept forgetting that it was okay not to want to spend every hour with my baby? That new moms didn't have to be euphoric all the time? When I was a burned-out bride-to-be, I remember how reassuring it was when Seth's mother pointed out that though weddings were wonderful, planning a party for 180 guests was no small task.

"I guess the kind of mother you have affects how you mother," I said. "I have to work at not feeling bad when I'm 'just' being a mom because my mom did so much more. Meanwhile other new mothers tell me they feel guilty whenever they do anything for themselves because their moms were totally devoted to raising children. Mothers are hard acts to follow either way."

"How is your mom?" Patty asked.

"Okay. She still cries a lot. I think she feels like she has this ghostly ménage à trois going on because she's reliving memories of Lewis and Dad." Poor Mom was raw and hurting. Seven years ago I was sad with her. This time I was mostly sad for her. "She said a lot of the sympathy notes say what a comfort it must be that Elizabeth is around, but that she thinks that's a heavy burden to lay on a baby. I sort of understand. Being a grandmother begins as a one-way love affair. But she also said she thinks of Elizabeth as a celebration — 'a continuation' — of her love with my dad, not with Lewis. I know Elizabeth can't be a cure-all. But I wish Mom would let her try to lift her spirits."

Patty nodded.

"She'll be more into grandmothering when Elizabeth is more of a person," I added. "I can't expect her to listen, rapt, to our adventures of going to buy a first pair of shoes, camera in hand, then being sent home because Elizabeth's feet were too small. Or to marvel just because Elizabeth has taken to emptying shelves, cruising around sofas, and giving people five."

Patty was quiet. "It's a tough one. It's a lot at once for both of you." She crouched in front of the stroller, turned to Elizabeth, and said, "Give me five."

Elizabeth did. Five and a great big smile.

A goose bit me. I was at Armonk's picturesque Wampus Pond, throwing bread to the ducks and geese, holding Elizabeth in my arms, and admiring the white gazebo and autumn red trees. The ducks were quacking, the geese were honking, Elizabeth was squealing, and all was well with the world.

Until I ran out of bread. Maybe it was because it was getting cold out. Maybe it was because it was midweek and no one else was feeding them. But the ducks and geese were not their fat and lazy selves. One particular stout and long-billed goose just wouldn't give up. He'd already had more than his share of stale bread, and when I ran out, he kept coming.

What was a mother to do?

I held Elizabeth close and the damn bird goosed me. He bit my thigh through my jeans and broke the skin, leaving an impressive black-and-blue.

It would fade. What worried me was this: what if Elizabeth had been older and had been standing on the ground? Would the goose have bitten her? Would she have developed goose and duck phobia? Turned against Mother Goose? Duck, Duck, Goose? Jemima Puddle-Duck? *Make Way for Ducklings?* All the little quackers that float in her bathtub and picture books?

A neighbor's dog snapped and snarled at Elizabeth that same week. It sent her into one of those sound-delayed crying jags that reminded me of how lightning precedes thunder. I soothed her, and I doubted she'd grow scared of dogs, though she might grow more wary, more respectful.

But at what age do such mini-traumas leave deeper impressions? I'm afraid of bees because as a child, I ran in the yard barefoot and kept stepping on them. I hope not to pass that fear on to Elizabeth. And I hope she doesn't pick up any phobias of her own.

Some might say Halloween has a scary side, but it's one reason why grown-ups should have children. I had more fun going door to door with Elizabeth on her first October 31 than I'd had on any Halloween since my own trick-or-treating days.

I wore a paint-speckled jumpsuit I'd bought at a street fair, and Elizabeth the ten-month-old sported a worn-out nightgown I had splattered à la Jackson Pollack. We both donned berets and went up and down our vertical neighborhood as twin *artistes*. Elizabeth loved standing before a closed door and helping me ring the bell. Who would answer? What would they look like? What would they give her? And where would Mommy take her next? The anticipation made her squeak and flail her arms.

I called Eric in Atlanta and told him about our adventures. He's not usually a killjoy, but his big-brother response was a bit deflating: "Yes, but when you two went around collecting candy," he wanted to know, "didn't everybody know it was for you?"

Rob and I always thought Elizabeth was a model baby. Now she was a baby model. Here's how it happened.

Strangers kept commenting on her pretty eyes and features. A few asked if she modeled. In a supermarket, one woman actually stopped me and said, "I have five grandkids and not one is as cute as your baby." I was appalled, but found myself gushing, thanking her and, yes, suddenly considering whether to send snapshots to modeling agencies.

In my youth I'd worked hard to earn seventy-five cents an hour baby-sitting. If Elizabeth could earn seventy-five dollars an hour modeling, maybe I should let her give it a try.

I didn't hire a photographer. I just went through our piles of pictures and made copies of an especially sweet one.

I glued the photos to pink cards with her name, weight, height, birth date, hair color, eye color, and a line about how she was flirtatious and flexible. I sent them to modeling agencies whose addresses I'd found in the yellow pages and in the Ross Reports, a brochure I'd bought at a bookstore.

And I waited.

Ford said no. Li'l Stars sent a form letter congratulating me since they receive "200–300 pictures per day" and said I could now buy their modeling book (twenty dollars) and schedule an interview on Staten Island (an hour away).

I figured I'd see what else came in the mail.

Two weeks passed and it looked as though Rascals Unlimited, Baby Wranglers Casting, and the other agencies weren't going to write back.

Then Wee Willy, the children's division of Wilhelmina, called. "Cute kid," Cami said.

"We think so."

"Can you bring her in this afternoon?"

"Sure."

"Three-thirty?"

"I'll be there."

I immediately went into stage-mom mode. I started thinking about how to arrange Elizabeth's nap schedule so she wouldn't be too tired. I wondered how to dress her. Whether I should teach her any new tricks. I worried that she might take a tumble and scratch herself before the interview. Or that, should all go well, she might grow up with a swelled head.

We arrived and Cami pronounced Elizabeth "adorable."

"She'll need a work permit, a social security number, a doctor's note, and a copy of her birth certificate," she said, then told me where to get the permit. "On Monday, there's a go-see for Enfamil." She wrote down the time and place and said there'd be other babies there.

Indeed there were. All plenty adorable.

I had painstakingly dressed Elizabeth, but the first thing I was asked to do was to strip her down to diapers. A woman then took the babies one by one to a white table where a photographer snapped Polaroids of them from front and behind.

"She's a doll," the woman said. But Elizabeth did as much fussing as chortling during her minute in the limelight. Then it was on to the next baby.

As I was dressing Elizabeth, I chatted with the other mothers. I joked that since I wasn't working on my career, I figured I'd work on Elizabeth's. Yet while these women clearly believed in baby modeling, I wasn't sure I did.

One woman spoke proudly of the shoots her baby had already done. Another moaned that this was her kid's seventh go-see and they had nothing to show for it.

Most of the babies were accompanied by their mothers, but a few were with nannies. That struck me as pushing it. Mothers, fathers, and kids shouldn't all be out earning a living, should they? At least Elizabeth was getting lots of mommy time and mommy kisses during our outing. And having people to see and places to go got us both outdoors — which was worth a lot, too.

"How'd you get started in this?" I asked. Most had stories like mine: strangers kept complimenting their child. One overweight woman said, "My mother did it for me when I was a kid. I enjoyed it and got a nest egg, too."

Did Enfamil sign us up? No.

But the next day, we were sent to a place called Mediagraphics. This time I dressed Elizabeth in comfortable clothes. The waiting room was full of Shirley Temple types, and Elizabeth and I played and read books until it was her turn. Then a stylist helped me dress her in a frilly outfit, spritzed her hair, wiped away her drool, and escorted us into the studio.

"Can she sit in a chair?"

"Not without falling off."

"Fine, just put her on the floor."

I put Elizabeth down, a Raffi tape played, and the photographer proceeded to make faces to get her to giggle. Elizabeth laughed, then got bored.

"Clap your hands," I said.

She clapped.

"Wave bye-bye."

She waved.

"How big is Elizabeth?" I asked.

She raised her hands high, then charged toward me as if to say, "What am I, a trained seal?"

I moved her back to the set and launched into a solo performance of "London Bridge Is Falling Down," "Heads, Shoulders, Knees, and Toes," and "In a Cottage in the Woods."

Two rolls of film later, they thanked us and had me sign a consent-and-release form. Elizabeth's fee for this shoot: sixty-five dollars, minus the agent's commission of 20 percent. A respectable beginning. But I was glad we had the next day off.

Bad enough that Elizabeth had once fallen from the sofa to the carpet. This time she rolled from the bed to the hardwood floor. Rob was on "cub patrol" when it happened and felt terrible. But so did I. I didn't want to win the Responsible Parent Award. I didn't want to be Martyr Mom. I wanted to feel that I could delegate the child care when I needed a break.

Once we'd determined that she was fine, that no goose eggs or horrible bruises were forthcoming, Rob, still contrite, showed me this passage from Spock's Baby Bible:

> A fall on the head is a common injury from the age when a baby can roll over (and thereby roll off a bed). A parent usually feels guilty the first time this happens. But if a child is so carefully watched that she *never* has an accident, she is being fussed over too much. Bones may be saved, but her character will be ruined.

"And Spock's your hero, don't forget."

"You're not in the dog house," I assured him. "But you have to keep an eye on her when you're in charge."

That night I lurched awake twice to grab what I imagined were Elizabeth's tiny toes going over the edge of the bed.

"This little piggy went to market," Rob began. "This little piggy stayed home. This little piggy had roast beef on a kaiser roll with Russian dressing. This little piggy had none on account of her diet. And this little piggy went wee wee wee all the way home."

"When I was a kid," I said, "I used to think the last piggy had been desperately crossing its legs and just couldn't hold it in anymore. I didn't realize it was oinking."

Beth and Ed were over and he, too, tried his hand at Elizabeth's foot. But Ed is a vegetarian, so when he got to the roast-beef toe, he said, "This little piggy had tofu."

Elizabeth beamed, and Beth gave her an early birthday gift: a tiny bomber jacket.

"Hey, did I tell you guys about my sperm test last week?" Ed asked.

Why, no. I freshened everybody's spiked eggnog.

"At the fertility clinic, they'd told us to 'refrain from having relations' for three days before my appointment. So when I went in, this nurse gave me a little jar — which was good because I was afraid she was going to give me a test tube and tell me to aim. Then she directed me to the bathroom."

"Were there dirty magazines?" Rob asked.

"Yeah, but they didn't have a very good selection — unless you had a thing for women with watermelon breasts."

"But you managed?" I inquired delicately.

"He managed," Beth said.

"I was under a lot of pressure. I didn't know if they were timing me. Or if when I handed over the jar, she'd say, 'That's all? Most men fill it to the top.'"

I looked at Elizabeth. Little pitchers have big ears, but I felt sure she was too young to be taking this in.

"Anyway," Ed continued, "they called yesterday and left a message on our machine saying my sperm are 'just fine.' The thing is, my second reaction was 'Just fine?' Not extraordinary? Not magnificent?"

Elizabeth had a doctor's appointment, too. Her one-year checkup. She weighed nearly twenty pounds and measured twenty-eight inches.

"She loves bath time but hates bedtime," I told Dr. Kahn. "She throws her bear and her pacifier out of the crib because she knows I'll retrieve them."

"My daughter used to do that. It's not a great game to encourage. How's she sleeping?"

"Fine." I considered telling him that sometimes I let her go to bed with a bottle. It always felt like I was doing us both a favor, but I knew bottles in bed were bad for her teeth, so decided not to confess. "She's been getting up around six o'clock," I said.

"What time does she go to sleep?"

"Around eight."

"That's ten hours. That's not unreasonable."

Maybe not, but when it was time for her wake-up call, Rob and I both hoped she'd ask for the other parent. At first I melted every time she called, "Mommy!" Now I was just as pleased when she began her day with "Daddy!"

I told Dr. Kahn that Elizabeth had had an upset stomach the previous week. He recommended the BRAT diet: bananas, rice, applesauce, and toast. As opposed, I wondered, to the toddler fish-and-chips diet, which consists of Pepperidge Farm Goldfish and Lays potato chips?

I mentioned that Elizabeth was doing some modeling and that although I had mixed feelings about it, it was fun for us to explore new neighborhoods and meet new people. "Yesterday, all she had to do was ride back and forth in a Cosco swing for a Toys 'Я' Us ad for *Parents,* and she made a hundred and fifty dollars."

"Not bad for someone who's not yet walking or talking," he said.

Course, having to look happy in a swing had been her easiest and best job yet. Having to look happy in a car seat that same week had been a whole 'nother story.

When we got home, Rob hugged Elizabeth and asked, "How's my birthday girl?"

"She got a clean bill of health." She looked back and forth at us and we reminisced about her first year.

"So," Rob asked, "when are we going to go for Baby Number Two?"

December and another round of holiday parties. It was hard to believe that last year's bowling ball was this year's one-year-old. A one-year-old who pushed around her oversize toy train and was steps away from walking. Who chomped on her pacifier as though it were the butt of a cigar: taking it out, turning it, admiring it, putting it back in. Who so loved seeing Labradors, poodles, and Scotties, that when I spotted one when I wasn't with her, I thought: a waste of a dog!

But there was something else different about the spirit of this Christmas. Last year, as a pregnant woman, I felt that everybody wished me well. This year I often felt judged. Everybody had an opinion about how I should be prioritizing my time, leading my life. And since I wasn't yet sure of my own choices, their opinions got to me.

At one of Rob's office parties, I spoke with a woman named Clara. "We've been very protective of our life-style," she said. "We agreed not to let things change after Jared came along."

"Really? We still travel and go out a lot, but by day, my life is dramatically different," I said.

"We've been looking for a school that can take him full-time," she went on, "but not a fancy school where the kids are all the same. He's twenty months and just started his interviews yesterday."

"We haven't thought about all that yet," I said, though the fear of God about private schools had been instilled in me since Day One.

"I like the idea of a school," she said, "because it would offer much more stimulation for Jared than if he just spent his days with the same person, shuttling back and forth to the park."

Wait a second. Had I missed something? Or had she just implied that a child not plunked into day care is being deprived of vital stimulation? That bathing a child in love during its formative years somehow holds it back? Full-time moms are

244

sometimes made to feel guilty about not making money or developing their own potential, but to turn around and accuse them of limiting their kids' development — this was too much.

Rob came over and he and I drifted toward the bar. "You two really hit it off," he observed.

"We despised each other," I corrected.

Motherhood, I was finding, was mined with Sensitive Issues. Back when we were all pregnant, we had been sisters. Now that we had babies, we were sometimes adversaries. Me, I was the mom in the middle. Tightroping between being a working and nonworking mother (talk about misnomers), I became everybody's confidante. Yet when homebound and office-bound women aimed potshots at each other, they sometimes nicked me in the crossfire.

"Some mothers feel they have to be there for every diaper change," a female stockbroker told me with derision. I nodded and smiled. But the next day, after changing Elizabeth, I noted that she immediately needed changing again. I was glad she wasn't at a school where they might not have noticed so quickly.

"How can she blithely trot off to her law firm each day?" a stay-at-home friend asked about one of our neighbors. "The nanny spends more time with their son than she does." I voiced agreement. But I knew the pull of the office.

"At first it's natural to be wrapped up in your baby," said a television producer, "but pretty soon you'll crave working again." Maybe she was right. But I didn't want to hear that my feelings were on a timer, that my rapture was a phase.

"At a party last night," complained a full-time mom, "this career woman was billing and cooing over her baby. Here I'd hired a sitter and was up for adult conversation, and this woman who never makes time for her kid comes off like Wonder Mom." I understood her point. But I understood the working mother, too.

A cousin told me about the birthday party she hosted. "You

know who I ended up entertaining? A dozen four-year-olds and their nannies. First I thought, 'What is wrong with this picture?' Then I thought, 'What is wrong with me?'"

When had things gotten so complicated? I felt I was straddling the fence between two camps. I didn't envy office moms or at-home moms. I envied women who were at peace, who weren't splintered by guilt and anxiety.

One of my editors told me I needed to get more child care: I had books to write.

Yes, but . . .

My agent advised, "Stay home if you possibly can. Kids will make you pay for every hour you neglect them. You can write later. I wish I had more memories of those early times."

Yes, but . . .

Strange. I'd been prepared for people to sniff at Elizabeth's budding (and short-lived) modeling career. I'd expected them to ask me about it, but roll their eyes on the sly. I wasn't surprised, for instance, when one of Rob's colleagues mentioned his nephew's part in a Broadway play and added, "the difference is that he *wants* to work."

But all this other static! All these attitudes! I usually enjoyed an easy rapport with women. Now I'd meet someone and our bristles might go up. We'd get self-righteous or defensive. Many of us were quietly afraid that we were abandoning our children or our careers, and neither choice was easy or without consequence.

I was lucky that, as a writer, I didn't have to make an either-or choice. I could work part-time and shift the balance periodically. Writing was my livelihood, but fortunately, we could manage if one or two years were less lively than usual.

Meantime, I was struggling to understand that different solutions work for different moms at different times. And that a mother's mental health matters, too: it's good for kids to have mothers who are happy.

Was I happy? I was pretty happy. I was getting more comfortable with my ambivalence. I was coming to realize that it might never go away. And I was beginning to accept that although I wasn't getting everything done — wasn't always even doing my best — I was doing what I could.

I was doing all I could.

I can't believe Elizabeth is a one-year-old," I told Jen.

"I can't believe I'm still single," she replied and laughed.

Apparently my daughter was marking time for all of us. She was now fourteen months old. She was not only walking, she was shaking her head no-no-no, unrolling toilet paper, playing "Ring Around the Rosey," leafing through lift-the-flap books, and standing on her head (with feet on the ground). She had not only said her first sentence, "Bye-bye, Daddy," but we'd already had our first conversation. It went something like this:

Scene: Mother walking with baby in backpack.

Mother: What does a cow say?

Baby: (*Silence*)

Mother: Mooo! What does a cat say?

Baby: (*Silence*)

Mother: Meow! What does a dog say?

Baby: (*After a pause*) Oof! Oof! Oof!

Sometimes, when my mind wasn't elsewhere, I'd look at Elizabeth, think how much fun she was, and wonder how I could have been so entranced with her back when she did so little. Then I'd realize that she was still hardly a rocket scientist, and that someday I might look at these wonder months and marvel that I found her captivating.

She also tried my patience. "Mom, forget this writing stuff. It's not worth it," she seemed to say as she emptied shelves of paperbacks into our bedroom wastebasket. When I ripped an article from a newspaper, she sometimes ripped a page from a picture book. I thought of the Phyllis Diller line, "Cleaning your house while your kids are still growing is like shoveling the walk before it stops snowing."

One day she insisted I try a spoonful of room-temperature peas. Do I have to? I wondered. It was one thing to share banana slices or yogurt, but pea mush? I opened my mouth and said "Thank you." But I draw the line at creamy turkey, I

248

thought, as I twisted the lids off turkey and carrot jars. Why did they make the jars so impossibly hard to open anyway? And if four and a half ounces of carrots provides only 4 percent of the recommended daily allowance of thiamine, where in heaven's name was my child supposed to get the other 96 percent?

Nancy's sons, Max and Harry, came to visit. Max, four, eyed a stack of cards. "Will you turn this into one hundred thousand dollars money?" he asked.

"What would you buy if I could?"

"Oh, shoes."

"What else?"

"Apple juice."

I poured him some juice, and Rob said, "You know, before we turn around, Elizabeth is going to be four."

"I know."

"Think when she's four her dolls will be having little domestic arguments?"

"Like what?"

"Like about alternate-side-of-the-street parking. You know: 'You move the car.' 'No, you.' 'No, I moved it yesterday.'"

Elizabeth was playing with the cordless phone. Not my favorite toy, but one that bought time in five-minute stretches. Max and Harry were building block towers. Brotherly love?

Rob and I began talking again about when to have a second baby. Although it had taken me a long time to feel ready to start a family, now that we had one baby, planning for a second seemed less of a leap. When Elizabeth was conceived, we'd felt alone among our peers. But her birth was like the first pop in the popcorn pot: it was quickly followed by others. Susan and Arlene had babies, and now Seth and Lucie were expecting. Lucie and I talked about nausea, nutrition, and nannies, and I was delighted that Elizabeth would have so many playmates.

Some people say second kids are easier. That instead of calling the doctor when your newborn sneezes, you just say, "Bless you." That instead of sterilizing a fallen pacifier, you just rinse it off — or insert it in your own mouth before inserting it in your baby's. But others warn that once you have a second child, you're embarrassed that you ever said you were busy when you had only one.

In a cab that week, my friend Judith advised me to wait another year before trying to conceive so that my kids would be three years apart. "That will give them time alone with you, and it will give you time to enjoy them."

No sooner did she hop out, however, than the cab driver interjected, "Nah. You want to have 'em close together. Get it over with."

I didn't know what I wanted. I didn't want to "get it over with" because, despite my back-and-forth feelings, I was relishing this period. Elizabeth brought us so much pleasure. I liked to think that my brothers and I had greeted our parents with smiles and giggles and a king and queen's welcome each day, too.

Current experts preached a three-year spacing between siblings, but I'd always imagined doing what my parents did, popping out kids one-two-three. Age gaps might be good for individuals, I reasoned, but for a family, wasn't it nice for kids to come one after another?

I'd always been very close to my brother Eric (just fourteen months older than I). And Mark (twenty-three months Eric's senior) and I were getting along better than ever because he'd moved back to New York — and because Elizabeth adored Uncle Marky. (The way to a mother's heart is through her kids.)

In theory, I was ready to go.

In reality, I was still catching my breath. Still working things out. Still tired.

Rob and I both had always felt we wanted at least two children, but he was tired, too. Sunday mornings weren't what they used to be, and this time he wasn't rushing me.

Yet though we didn't feel ready, this time we also knew we

probably never would. So slowly slowly we came to decide to go for round two. We loved Elizabeth and hoped to get lucky again.

"Do you know how crazy it's going to be with two whirling dervishes around here?" I asked. We watched as our daughter, on her third or fourth wind, ricocheted around the room.

"Totally out of control," Rob answered. "Double trouble. But that's why you have a second child — so someday you can look exasperated, put your hands on your hips, and yell, 'KIDS!'"

At a year and four months, Elizabeth gave up her pacifier. I thought we'd have an endless struggle. I thought she was as attached to her piece of rubber as Bart Simpson's T.V. sister Maggie is to hers. But when I misplaced Elizabeth's favorite and offered an alternate, she summarily rejected it. *And went to sleep anyway!*

That was the good news. The bad news was that now when she woke up at night, I sometimes had to sing songs or offer a bottle instead of just jiggling the plug. And when she fussed during the day, there was no quick fix. Which meant I could no longer take her everywhere and anywhere.

To museums, for instance. Elizabeth had liked the cows, faces, and colors of a Warhol exhibit. She'd liked the horses, dresses, and babies of a Velázquez exhibit. But the Canalettos at the Met were a challenge. Just water and boats. More water, more boats.

She grew suddenly impatient. Loudly impatient. A crinkled-up woman said, "This is not a nursery. Your baby is annoying everybody." I shh'd Elizabeth, squinted at the woman, and wished I had the guts to reply, "You were young once, too — or perhaps not."

I didn't and we left. Outside it was raining. And I hadn't brought an umbrella or a plastic stroller canopy.

"Damn!" I muttered, and studied the downpour.

"Duck!" Elizabeth shrieked, and pointed to a pigeon.

A cab pulled up. I grabbed Elizabeth and made a run for it. A man I hadn't seen reached the door at the exact moment I did.

"Ladies first?" I said.

"Not today," he retorted, and opened the door as I was fiddling with the stroller.

"You're kidding." I was dumbfounded. I love New York. When someone bad-mouths my city, I fiercely defend it. New York is a great place to be a culture vulture and to people watch.

Where else can you go to the park and see ferrets on leashes, cockatoos on shoulders, pet monkeys, and pet pythons? Where else can you order in Thai food, pasta primavera, or pastrami sandwiches at midnight? Still, there were days when I had to put down my Pollyanna shield and reckon with the rudeness.

"I'm not kidding," the man said and climbed in. "C'mon, Jerry," he called to his friend.

Jerry stood under an umbrella a few yards away and, bless him, said, "Let the lady have the cab."

The man got out grumbling. "Thanks," I mumbled, and Elizabeth and I headed home under the April shower.

On my answering machine was a message from Wee Willy. I dialed their number and, when Elizabeth complained, I placated her by doling out Gerber meat sticks one at a time — a practice that horrified Ed, the tofu-eater.

"A magazine saw photos of Elizabeth and wants her to appear on their cover," said Noreen.

"That's great!" I was feeling better already.

"Wait. It's a small magazine and they'll pay only forty dollars."

"That might be okay."

"The shoot is in Jersey City."

"Oh." I'd promised myself that if Elizabeth's modeling ever became work instead of fun for either of us, we'd drop out.

"It gets better. They want to dress her as a boy, in a sailor suit."

"Noreen," I said, "Maybe you should make someone else's day."

I could handle stylists gussying Elizabeth up with hair bows, lacy anklets, and colorful bracelets. I didn't object much when they tried to bribe her with Cheerios. I didn't even mind when nineteen-year-old French models got to pose as her mother. But I'd said no once to a blow dryer and curling iron. And I could say it again to cross-dressing in Jersey City.

Summertime, and the living was easy. More or less.

At the playground, Elizabeth, now one and a half, made a beeline for the big slide. I watched, heart in throat, as she clambered up the steps. When she reached the top, I was terrified. I didn't know whether to stay where I was, ready to catch her if she fell backward, or run to the front, ready to catch her if she pushed off. "Mark, Set, Go!" Elizabeth called, and I dashed to the front, extended my arms, and caught her speeding body — just in time.

At home I grilled Rob. "What did you teach her?"

"What?"

"The playground. We used to sit and swing and watch people. Now she's a daredevil and I'm scared out of my mind." Gone were the days of parenthood as spectator sport.

"You mean the slide? She's great at the slide. She loves the slide."

"Yeah, but I hate it."

It was all very well that Rob looked after Elizabeth on occasional weekend mornings. But his idea of child care sometimes meant teaching his daughter dangerous playground stunts. Or staying glued to Mr. Rogers's interview of pianist André Watts long after Elizabeth had wandered away. Or showing her how to jump into puddles because, he reasoned, "Life is too short not to." Yet I was always the one left to deal with the wet sneakers.

Granted, I was thankful for the every-once-in-a-while morning breaks. Some husbands never help their wives. But then why do we always use the word "help"? Both parents' names go on birth certificates, don't they?

Recently, after playing with Elizabeth all morning, I handed her to Rob, dirty diaper and all. He whisked her away, singing "Take Me Out to the Ball Game." An older friend was visiting and whispered, "He's wonderful with the baby." I agreed. But sometimes I thought *I* should be canonized. How come dads get the same credit for quality minutes as moms do for quality hours?

Even without encouragement, Elizabeth was becoming a wild child. She'd wake up indignant, shouting, "No more nap!" She'd move chairs and scramble up them. Run penguinlike and fall on her face. Unwind cassettes and rearrange drawers. Turn round and round until she made herself dizzy. Attempt somersaults. Ram her wheelbarrow into the T.V. and say, "'Scuse me, Mr. Rogers." Climb on benches and say, "Be careful!" Stand in her high chair and say, "Sit down!" Approach elevator doors and say, "No, no, no!"

Once she even jumped from her crib. It frightened all three of us, and we surrounded the area with blankets. She never did it again.

When Elizabeth wasn't worrying me, she was melting my heart. When I said her bath was hot, she blew on it. When I wore a Woody Jackson T-shirt with a farm scene on it, she pointed to the cow and mooed. She hummed "Frère Jacques" and "Skip to My Lou." She said "More?" whenever we finished a story or song or bowl of cereal. She loved identifying eyebrows and belly buttons. Thanks to Matilde, she could count in Spanish — though not always in any particular order. And she was so tender and affectionate with Teddy that I thought someone should write *The Sensuous Baby*.

But she was not a baby anymore. She was a little girl.

Elizabeth was putting on and taking off her party shoes as Jenny, the baby-sitter, was reading to her. When had I become a mother? I remembered reading books to children when I was a baby-sitter. I even remembered baby-sitters reading books to me.

"Here's the number of our pediatrician," I told Jenny.

"Dr. Kahn!" Jenny exclaimed. "He's my doctor!" Suddenly fourteen seemed younger than I'd thought.

I offered final instructions, kissed Elizabeth good-bye, locked the door, and listened to hear if she would cry. All was quiet as I stepped into the elevator.

Inside, a little boy I'd never seen asked, "Where are you going?"

An out-of-line question, but one I was proud to answer. "I'm going to meet Raffi. Do you like Raffi?"

He nodded, wide-eyed. "I have his tapes," he said and studied me with awe.

"His publisher is throwing him a party." For the benefit of the grown-ups, I added, "Raffi is to kids today what Captain Kangaroo was to us."

Frankly, I was thrilled when *Redbook* passed the invitation along. Sure, there were days when I thought that if I had to listen to "Down by the Bay" one more time, I'd go screaming into the Hudson. But mostly I felt only gratitude toward the bearded Canadian whose gentle voice could get Elizabeth to go from sobbing to dancing in a matter of minutes.

I reached the United Nations Plaza and entered the elevator. Inside stood Raffi. "You're Raffi," I blurted. "You're the man we've come to see."

"And you?" he asked, extending his hand.

"Carol Weston." He graciously introduced his two escorts.

"My daughter loves you!" I gushed. "I love you!"

Years ago I'd met Paul Newman and interviewed Joanne

Woodward, and even then I don't think I came off quite so star-struck, so stupid-sounding. I pressed on. "The first thing my daughter says in the morning is 'Raffi.' And whenever she gets restless in the car, we put on your music, and she hums and sings and bounces along. You're magic!"

He smiled and we stepped out onto the twelfth floor. A publicist handed me a name tag. Raffi waved his away. "People will have to figure out who I am by process of elimination."

On the table were complimentary copies of his new book, *Everything Grows*. I took one and got out the two I'd brought from home, *Five Little Ducks* and *Wheels on the Bus*. He seemed to be stalling before entering the party room, so I said, "Would you mind signing these?"

"I'd be glad to, Carol." Granted, I'd just introduced myself, and granted, my name was written in block letters on my chest. But I was still impressed that he used it.

In a flash, he'd signed his name twice. (Like Cher and Madonna, he isn't burdened with excess letters.) On the third book, I grew bold. "Could you add, 'For Elizabeth'?"

"For Elizabeth," he added.

Boy was I pleased!

We walked into the party and he was swallowed up by admirers. I helped myself at the buffet, then sat down with some publicity people. We were talking about book-party food when one of their colleagues rushed over. "He's sitting down signing books. A line is forming!" She seemed alarmed. "We want people to talk to him, not ask for autographs."

One of the publicists tried to discourage the fans, but they didn't budge. I didn't blame them, and I felt a retroactive pang of guilt for having accosted Raffi at the door. I decided to be helpful and went over to ask him if he'd had dinner.

"May I fix you a plate?"

"That would be nice."

"Are you a vegetarian?" I figured a man who sings about cows, pigs, and ducks just might be.

"I don't eat meat or chicken, but anything else would be fine."

"I'll be right back." I heaped his plate high with shrimp, hummus, cannelloni, cheese, bread, and vegetables.

"Here you go."

"Thank you."

"Hey, I owed you one for the autographs." If Elizabeth had been older, I would have brought her along. Instead, I had to hope she'd someday appreciate her growing number of autographed books: *The Very Hungry Caterpillar* signed by Eric Carle, *Eloise* signed by Hilary Knight, *Babar* signed by Laurent de Brunhoff, and now the Raffi books. "Besides," I added, "you made my night."

Raffi thanked me again and kissed my cheek. Had I been ten, I'd have vowed never to wash it again.

On the bus uptown, I thought of his lyric, "All I really need is a song in my heart, food in my belly, and love in my family." Pure schmaltz, but thinking of Elizabeth, I felt oddly moved. I was surprised to realize that my ever-growing list of heroes seemed to include not only my old standbys — Gabriel García Márquez, Mel Gibson, and Dr. Spock — but now that pied-piping music-making sandbox superstar, Raffi Cavoukian.

Buddy Holly was crooning "Maybe Baby" on the stereo. Elizabeth turned up the volume. I turned it down.

My daughter was pushing two and her taste in music had expanded to include Burl Ives, Sharon, Lois & Bram, James Taylor, early Beatles, and rock 'n' roll hits from "La Bamba" to "Let's Go to the Hop."

Lucie and I were playing with her new baby, my godson Marc. "Niiiice baby," Elizabeth said and stroked his head. She liked Marc — so long as *I* didn't pay too much attention to him. She tapped my arm and, just to set the record straight, announced, "That's Libeebee's mommy."

"I'm Elizabeth's mommy," I confirmed. Reassured, she went back to her Cheerios, carefully setting aside all the closed ones and broken ones. She was a born quality-control expert. And I was never far behind with the Dustbuster.

"I know I love Marc," Lucie said, "because in the park, a bee landed on his carriage and instead of going screaming off in the other direction, I stuck around until it buzzed away."

"I know I love Elizabeth because I don't hold it against her that she and Teddy have make-out sessions, whereas I usually have to beg for kisses and hugs." Elizabeth had grown so attached to Teddy that we didn't dare wash him except at night — at which time we'd quietly kidnap him from her crib, run him through the fastest washer-dryer cycle, then replace him as quickly as possible.

I poured Lucie some orange juice with seltzer water. "Want to know a secret?"

Her eyes lit up. "You're pregnant?"

"You got it!"

"Wheeeeeee! That's great! That's so great!"

"I'm due in June. It took five months this time. Last time it took five minutes."

"That is so great! I'm so excited for you! Wait until I tell

Seth!" Lucie gave me an effusive hug. Then she looked serious. "How are you guys going to manage?"

"Good question. I hear bunk beds are key. The first years are going to be tough. Elizabeth is good at sharing toys, but sharing Mommy is going to be another story. I mean, I wouldn't like it if Rob came home and said, 'Carol, meet Wanda. I'm going to be her husband now, too.'"

Lucie laughed. "I have a friend who just had a second baby and says she feels this wonderful completeness. She also says you're not nearly as anxious the second time. You're an expert instead of a novice."

"That's good to hear. I have a friend who just had a second baby and says she feels like he's her secret lover because whenever the older brother leaves the room, she showers the new one with kisses. She says the hardest thing about having a second kid is watching the first one go from a sweetheart to a monster."

When Elizabeth turned two, I took her out of modeling. It had been an interesting experience and she had acquired a small portfolio of ads as well as a hummingbird-size nest egg. But now that I was pregnant again, I was tired. There was no sleeping in or taking naps this time around, and carrying Elizabeth's stroller up and down subway steps was too much.

Besides, the agencies suddenly expected more than a pretty face. They expected my daughter to act. To roll a ball or hold another child's hand or walk through a tire simply because they said to. To bond with Big Bird — touching his beak while smiling at the camera. For a Johnson & Johnson shampoo ad, they expected her not to cry when they glopped lather on her hair. No More Tears? Elizabeth bawled.

At our last shoot, she insisted on trying to put on the shoes herself, which took twenty minutes. Then a stylist got her dressed, but when I tried to set her in the middle of the set, she clung to me. She wouldn't even put down her landing gear. Who needed it?

"We're booking out," I told Cami at Wee Willy. "She's not at a cooperative age and I'm not willing to fight with her." In talks and articles, I always told mothers of teens to choose their quarrels well. I was ready to practice what I preached. "Besides," I added, "I'm pregnant again."

Pregnant again. It felt good to be pregnant again. I didn't pat my tummy as much as last time. Didn't look into the mirror or crystal ball as often. Didn't rush into maternity clothes. And didn't get quite as big a kick out of getting big and getting kicked. As far as not lifting heavy objects, I had Elizabeth to tote around.

But it felt good to be pregnant again.

To be in a family way.

To know that in a few months we'd have another lovable baby who would someday smile, laugh, walk, talk — and even love us back.

Having a child is great. Being great with child is too.

This is how J. M. Barrie's *Peter Pan and Wendy* begins:

All children, except one, grow up. They soon know that they will grow up, and the way Wendy knew was this. One day when she was two years old she was playing in a garden, and she plucked another flower and ran with it to her mother. I suppose she must have looked rather delightful, for Mrs Darling put her hand to her heart and cried, "Oh, why can't you remain like this for ever!" This was all that passed between them on the subject, but henceforth Wendy knew that she must grow up. You always know after you are two. Two is the beginning of the end.

The beginning of the end. The end of the beginning. I wanted Elizabeth to grow up so that I could read Barrie's whole book to her. But I also wished she could stay a spirited little toddler forever.

We loved our pint-size sophisticate, our urbanite in overalls. She held court in elevators, flirted with doormen, hailed cabs, ran down ramps at the Guggenheim, and thrilled at the sound of a siren. Rob and I were both brought up in suburbia, but Elizabeth preferred pâté to applesauce, Zabar's to just any deli. She was a regular at the Children's Museum of Manhattan and the Museum of Natural History. Thanks to gifts and hand-me-downs, she had a wardrobe that put mine to shame. She liked piling on necklaces and wearing several hats at a time. And she loved starring in the outgoing message of our answering machine — she'd often put her own singular spin on classic tunes, such as "Mary Had a Little Yam," "Sing a Song of Penguins," and "Old MacDonald Had a Cow."

She was also becoming a miniature mommy. She liked to diaper Teddy, to push him in her baby carriage, to offer food, drink, a toothbrush. She was solicitous about other toys, too.

When a helium balloon floated to the ceiling, she looked at me and asked, "Balloon bumped her head?"

Meantime, I had started working about thirty hours a week. When Elizabeth turned two, and I knew I'd soon have another newborn in the house, I decided it was time for us both to declare a little independence. She'd enjoy having a life outside the home, and I'd enjoy having time to work hard before the next baby arrived, and before I started cocooning again. I had finally come to understand why my mother needed both the paycheck and the pulse of the office. And I had realized at last that while I loved being a mom, I didn't want — or have — to give up my previous identity.

Elizabeth continued spending some mornings with Matilde, and now spent two days in day care. She no longer cried when I left her there and no longer made me feel I'd rescued her when I picked her up. She had also graduated from bottle to cup. And from crib to big-girl bed.

She was growing up. Yet at almost two and a half, she was still a sweet innocent. One morning we passed a homeless man wrapped in a blanket. "Shhh! Man sleeping," she said. A homeless woman tickled Elizabeth's toes in her stroller, and she laughed merrily. One night she woke up from a dream and, still asleep herself, asked, "Where cookies? Where juice?" Even her nightmares were painted in pastels.

She had a lot to learn about the world and about her family. Sometimes I'd ask her what was inside my belly and she'd brighten and say, "Baby inside." But then she'd pat her own belly and say, "Baby inside Libeebee's belly, too."

Other times she'd point to our framed photos and would identify everybody, unaware of how much that meant to me. "That's Mommy, that's Daddy, that's Uncle Marky, that's Eric, that's Cynthia, that's Grandmary, that's Mommy's Daddy." Hear that? I'd think. I'm keeping my promise, Dad. Your memory lives on.

What would Elizabeth's first memory be? Was it already en-

graved? Or will it come very soon, when she meets her brother
or sister? It was hard to believe that so far her trips and tumbles
may have left no traces. That her sunny days may have marked
her personality but not her memory.

Occasionally it seemed that as I grew bigger and bigger, she
regressed more and more. By the time I was nine months pregnant, we'd kissed millions of invisible boo-boos and endured
numerous irrational tantrums. Sometimes she'd fake-cry while
studying herself in the mirror. Sometimes, just to be contrary,
she'd matter-of-factly drop God-knows-what in a full wastebasket and announce "Garbage."

One morning on the street, she had a total breakdown because Teddy was at home (where Teddy nearly always stayed). I
assumed passersby took me for a shrew, but one gentleman was
kind enough to pause and smile knowingly. "Two?" he asked.

Two indeed. At times Rob and I joked about sitting Elizabeth
down and saying, "Look, honey, this just isn't working out."
But her summer storms blew over quickly.

"You know the poem," I asked him,

> "There was a little girl
> Who had a little curl
> Right in the middle of her forehead,
> And when she was good,
> She was very, very good,
> But when she was bad she was horrid?"

"What about it?"

"Did you know Longfellow wrote it?"

"No," Rob said. "But I bet he had a two-year-old daughter at
the time."

That morning I dragged Elizabeth home, handed her Teddy,
turned on her favorite video — Disney's *Heigh-Ho* — and
seized the opportunity to snip her finger- and toenails. When
Winnie the Pooh sang, "I'm short and fat and proud of that," I
rubbed my own round belly. Elizabeth stroked my hair. "Niiiice

Mommy," she said and beamed angelically. Dr. Jekyll and Ms. Hyde.

"Do you want some orange juice or apple juice?" I asked.

"Orange juice or apple juice?" she replied.

My father-in-law called and we talked about business. "Say, 'I love you, Poppa,'" I prompted, and Elizabeth took the phone and said, "I love you, Poppa."

"Ken, I know you have a heart of stone," I said, "but doesn't that chip away at it a little bit?" I was reminded of when we three took a walk and she caught him off guard by reaching up and grabbing hold of his hand.

"Kids should be locked up in the closet until they're old enough to read Greek," Ken answered. He had a reputation to uphold.

"Grandmary coming?" Elizabeth asked me.

She was looking forward to a visit with my mother. So was I. Mom and I were both on a more even keel, and it seemed that just as I began to expect less, she began to offer more. "I bought her a kangaroo with a baby in its pouch," she said on the phone. "I couldn't resist. Should I give it to her now or wait until the baby is born?"

"Might as well wait," I said. "Could be any day now."

And that's where things stand. Baby Number Two is due in two weeks. It would be great to have another girl because we adore our first girl. It would be great to have a boy because then we'd have one of each. Both grandmothers are on call again, waiting for news and waiting to help.

Patty will be the godmother and Ed will be the godfather. He and Beth are not yet expecting, but they've learned, as her doctor put it, that her "plumbing is in order," and that they're not "allergic to each other." So time will tell. Amazingly, many of our other friends are already pregnant again: Arlene, Susan, Lucie.

It's odd to be a mother who has never broken water or had a

contraction. To be, well, a virgin at all this. My ob/gyns are talking about a VBAC — vaginal birth after cesarean. They're hoping to deliver the new baby the old-fashioned way, and I'm hoping to help them, breath by breath.

Last week, at the ob/gyn's, I fell asleep in their armchair. I was dreaming I was at a beach trying to keep up with two rambunctious kittens. Nurse Liz called my name, and I awakened with a start. "You can always tell the pregnant mothers with toddlers at home," she said. "They're the ones who nod off in the waiting room."

Today I brought Elizabeth along for my now-weekly appointment. We listened to the fetal heartbeat, and when the nurse put away the doppler, Elizabeth protested. "One more time?" she asked.

When we were ready to leave, I snapped up her jacket and threw on mine. "Zip Mommy's jacket?" she said.

"Good idea, honey." I felt the other pregnant women study us as Elizabeth coaxed the zipper over my prodigious belly, over the infant whose name we would soon know.

"Good luck!" I called and took my daughter's hand. "The hours are long, but the rewards are tremendous." I knew *I'd* need luck, too. Each day and each year would present new hurdles.

Yet on the way home, I found myself once again feeling proud, excited, and nervous. This time I knew about the pain of childbirth. But I also knew about the joy of children. The motherhood mosaic has pieces that are dark and dull, but it's a work that shines.

I pat my belly, I put my arm around my daughter, and I am so happy that Rob and I began all this over three years ago. And that now, in two weeks, baby will make four.

A child for each hand.

A child for each parent.

A family.